ATI TEAS 7th EDITION EXAM PREP:

Disclaimer: This book is not affiliated with, sponsored by, or endorsed by the Assessment Technologies Institute (ATI). All test names and other trademarks are the property of the respective trademark holders. None of the trademark holders are affiliated with this book or endorse this specific product.

The material in this book is intended for educational purposes only. It is designed to provide accurate information in regard to the subject matter covered. However, it is provided with the understanding that the publisher and author are not engaged in rendering legal, accounting, or other professional advice. If such advice or other expert assistance is required, the services of a competent professional should be sought.

While every effort has been made to ensure the accuracy of the information presented in this book as of the publication date, the author and publisher make no representations or warranties with respect to the accuracy or completeness of the contents of this work and specifically disclaim all warranties, including without limitation warranties of fitness for a particular purpose.

The strategies, tips, and techniques suggested in this book are the author's own and do not guarantee a successful outcome on the ATI TEAS exam. The exam's structure and content are subject to changes by its conducting body, and readers are advised to ensure they are referring to the latest version of the exam and using the most up-to-date study materials.

The author and publisher shall not be liable for any loss of profit or any other commercial damages, including but not limited to special, incidental, consequential, or other damages.

PAGE 2 INTRODUCTION:

PAGE 7 READING SECTION:

PAGE 15 MATHEMATICS SECTION:

PAGE 26 SCIENCE SECTION:

PAGE 35 ENGLISH AND LANGUAGE USAGE SECTION:

PAGE 45 EXAM PREP SECTION: (1,200+ Practice Exam Questions and Answers)

INTRODUCTION:

Ready to unlock the mysteries of human anatomy, algebraic equations, cellular biology, and the intricacies of the English language? It might sound like a daunting task, but rest assured - this journey is yours to embark upon, and we are here to guide you through it.

In your hands, you hold more than just a study guide. This is a roadmap, a steadfast companion prepared to accompany you through the vast landscapes of the Assessment Technologies Institute (ATI) Test of Essential Academic Skills (TEAS), 7th Edition.

But let's be honest; this voyage won't always be smooth sailing. There will be concepts that challenge you, questions that may stump you, moments when you might stumble. But remember - it's okay. It's all part of the journey. Failure is not a roadblock, but a stepping stone to success, a teacher that shows us where we need to focus our efforts.

So, if you're feeling apprehensive about the science section, don't worry. We'll delve into the marvelous complexity of the human body, journeying through the intricacies of the cardiovascular, digestive, nervous, and other vital systems. We'll decode the building blocks of life in cell biology, and wrestle with the engaging challenges of chemistry.

If math has you feeling uneasy, fret not. We're here to demystify numbers, transforming them from foes to allies. From basic arithmetic to real-world problems involving percentages, ratios, and algebra, we'll navigate these numerical seas together.

If reading comprehension or English language usage has you on edge, we've got you covered. We will explore how to infer meaning from texts, analyze information, and express your thoughts clearly and correctly. It's all about empowering you with the skills to master the English language in all its beauty.

This guide is more than a compilation of facts and figures. It's a tool for encouragement and empowerment, carefully designed to help you rise above your fears, transform your failures into stepping stones, and focus your energies on achieving your dream of acing the TEAS exam. It's time to pick up your metaphorical rocks and take aim at the obstacles in your path.

Your dream is within reach, and this guide is here to prove it to you. So, let's step into this journey together and embark on this wonderful voyage of learning and discovery. Your TEAS exam success story starts now. Let's write it together.

Cracking the code of the TEAS exam, you ask? Consider it done. The Test of Essential Academic Skills, fondly known as the TEAS, is a pivotal point on the pathway to healthcare and nursing programs across the United States. With this test, potential students showcase their proficiency and understanding in areas deemed necessary for success in the health science field. This trial by knowledge is conducted under the watchful eyes of the Assessment Technologies Institute (ATI).

One might picture the TEAS exam as a four-course academic banquet, each dish representing a key area of study: Reading, Mathematics, Science, and English and Language Usage. This isn't your usual quick meal - you'll have 209 minutes to savor these four courses, comprising 170 questions in total.

Starting with the Reading course, it whets the appetite with a variety of text types. With 53 questions served in 64 minutes, you'll engage with passages and documents, graphs, and charts. But the key here isn't just about understanding the words. It's about digging beneath the surface - finding main ideas, discerning the author's intent, making inferences. You'll interpret, analyze, and evaluate to navigate this section.

Next comes the Mathematics course, a mix of 36 questions spread over 54 minutes. Here, your ability to play with numbers and your grasp of basic operations, fractions, percentages, algebra, and data interpretation is on the menu. Mathematics is the universal language, and this course allows you to speak it fluently.

Then we move onto the Science course, perhaps the main course for those heading towards healthcare. This section immerses you in the wonders of the natural world, from human anatomy to cell biology, and from genetics to chemistry. Over 63 minutes, you'll traverse 53 questions designed to probe your scientific knowledge and reasoning skills.

Last but not least is the English and Language Usage course. In this section, spanning 28 questions in 28 minutes, your mastery of the English language comes to the fore. Conventions of standard English, vocabulary acquisition, language and word usage - it's all about ensuring clear and effective communication.

This journey through the TEAS exam might sound demanding, even a little intimidating, but remember - this guide, this roadmap, is here to accompany you every step of the way. It's designed not merely to assist you in understanding the layout of the TEAS exam, but to offer in-depth knowledge, strategies, and practice to ensure that you are fully prepared to excel in each of these areas. Your success is our mission, and we're here to make it happen. So, shall we begin?

An important milestone on the road to a career in healthcare, the TEAS exam wields substantial influence over your admission into nursing programs. But why does it hold such a distinguished status? The reasons are as numerous as the questions on the test itself.

Firstly, the TEAS offers an unbiased lens through which schools view prospective students. By distilling academic potential into quantifiable scores, it delivers a common measure that cuts across differing educational backgrounds. A high score on the TEAS is a strong indicator of your readiness for the rigors of a nursing program. It reflects your ability to absorb, integrate, and apply the academic knowledge that forms the bedrock of healthcare professions.

Secondly, nursing programs are not just looking for knowledge, but also for aptitude. They are on the lookout for individuals who can handle the diverse challenges of the healthcare world. The TEAS, through its broad assessment of reading, mathematics, science, and English language skills, provides a snapshot of your intellectual versatility. It underscores your potential to juggle multiple disciplines - a skill that will be invaluable in the multidisciplinary world of nursing.

Thirdly, nursing is a demanding field. The robust curriculum, intense clinical experiences, and high stakes of patient care require resilience and steadfast commitment. Completing the TEAS test and achieving a high score demonstrates your dedication and serious intent to the nursing program of your choice. It shows that you're not just willing to meet the challenges of nursing education, but that you are ready to excel.

Finally, the TEAS exam not only opens the door to a nursing program but also sets the foundation for your nursing licensure. Many states consider your TEAS score during the nursing licensure process, making it a critical stepping stone on your path to becoming a registered nurse.

The TEAS is more than just a test—it's a passport to your nursing career. A strong score not only improves your chances of admission into your dream nursing program but also signals your readiness for the demanding journey ahead. It demonstrates your commitment, resilience, and potential to succeed in a field that's as challenging as it is rewarding. Prepare for it well, and it will undoubtedly open doors to a promising future in healthcare.

Let look at the **structure of the exam**. Think of it as a well-orchestrated symphony, composed of four major movements, each representing a specific academic discipline: Reading, Mathematics, Science, and English & Language Usage. Like any symphony, each part is unique, yet they come together to create a harmonious and comprehensive piece.

First, the "Reading Movement" comes into play. You will face 45 questions timed for 55 minutes. This section gauges your comprehension skills, like summarizing texts, locating specific information, and drawing conclusions. It also probes your ability to understand written directions, interpret graphical information, and evaluate the author's purpose and viewpoint.

Next, the "Mathematics Movement" enters the symphony. In this section, you will be given 38 questions to solve in 57 minutes. The questions test your understanding of numbers and algebra, including converting fractions, decimals, and percentages, solving equations, and handling real-world problems that involve proportions, ratios, rates of change, and the interpretation of data.

Then, we proceed to the "Science Movement," which comprises 50 questions you will address within 60 minutes. This section is designed to assess your knowledge in human anatomy & physiology, biology, and chemistry. You'll answer questions about body systems, cell structure, genetic material, atomic structure, chemical reactions, and the properties of solutions.

Finally, the "English & Language Usage Movement" concludes the symphony. In this section, you will respond to 37 questions within a 37-minute timeframe. This section measures your understanding of English language conventions, knowledge of language, and your ability to use language and vocabulary to express ideas effectively.

It's crucial to understand that these aren't random questions. They're designed with a purpose, each working in tandem to provide a thorough evaluation of your academic preparedness for a healthcare career. As you embark on this journey through the TEAS exam, remember that each question is a stepping stone on the path to your dream nursing program. Your ability to navigate these four sections with skill and confidence is the key to unlocking your future in healthcare.

Navigating the sea of **scoring and interpretation in the TEAS exam** may appear daunting, but let's break it down to simpler elements. Remember, each ripple you create in this sea leads you closer to your desired nursing program.

Now, the TEAS exam consists of 170 questions. However, in this universe of questions, 150 are scored and 20 are unscored pretest questions used for test development purposes. This implies that your score is based only on those 150 questions.

Each of these 150 questions carries equal weight, meaning each correct response contributes equally to your overall score. Here's where the magic begins: instead of raw scores, the TEAS uses a scaled scoring system. This method ensures fairness and consistency across different versions of the test.

You will receive a composite score, which represents your overall performance, and individual scores for each of the four content areas: Reading, Mathematics, Science, and English & Language Usage. These scores are represented as percentages. For instance, if you answer 90 out of 150 scored questions correctly, your composite score is 60%.

But how do you interpret this? Your score gets classified into performance bands: Developmental, Basic, Proficient, Advanced, and Exemplary. Each band reflects a certain level of preparedness for nursing or allied health education.

Interpreting your score isn't about scrutinizing a single number. Instead, it's about understanding the story that your performance tells across the four sections. Each score uncovers your strengths and weaknesses, providing a roadmap to your future learning journey.

In the grand scheme of the TEAS, your score isn't just a statistical measure; it is a reflection of your diligence, perseverance, and the potential to thrive in a healthcare career. It's the numerical encapsulation of your efforts, the very key that opens the door to your nursing aspirations.

Embracing the day of your TEAS exam can seem nerve-racking. But with a well-structured plan and mindset, it can turn into an empowering experience. Here are

1. **The Early Bird Catches the Worm**: Arrive early at the test center. This gives you ample time to settle down, adapt to your surroundings, and mentally prepare for the exam.
2. **Familiarity Breeds Confidence**: Be aware of the test format, the types of questions, and the time allowed for each section. This helps prevent surprises on test day.
3. **Equip Yourself**: Bring the necessary items such as your admission ticket, valid photo ID, and pencils. But remember, leave behind any materials not allowed in the test center.
4. **Dress for Success**: Choose comfortable clothing. Test centers can be chilly, so consider dressing in layers to accommodate the room temperature.
5. **Your Body, Your Ally**: Ensure you're well-rested, hydrated, and nourished. A good night's sleep, a light meal, and plenty of water can significantly influence your performance.
6. **Read and Heed**: Carefully read all instructions before starting each section of the test. Misreading can lead to mistakes even when you know the correct answer.
7. **Time is Gold**: Keep an eye on the clock. Try to maintain a steady pace and avoid spending too much time on a single question. Remember, each question counts the same towards your score.
8. **Think Positive, Be Positive**: Approach the exam with a positive attitude. This can help reduce anxiety and increase your ability to focus. Remember, you've prepared for this.
9. **Pace, Don't Race**: Don't rush through the questions. Read each one thoroughly, and be sure to understand what it's asking before answering.
10. **Embrace the Breaks**: Utilize the provided breaks wisely. Use this time to rest your mind, stretch, hydrate, and mentally prepare for the next section.

Remember, test day is a culmination of all your preparation. Treat it as an opportunity to display your knowledge and skills. You're not just taking a test; you're taking a significant step on your journey to becoming a healthcare professional.

READING SECTION:

The Reading section of the TEAS exam is designed to assess a student's ability to comprehend, interpret, and apply information from various types of text. It forms a fundamental pillar of the test, emphasizing the essential role reading comprehension plays in nursing and healthcare. The section comprises 53 questions and is allotted 64 minutes for completion, with the aim of evaluating the ability of candidates to effectively process written information, a skill crucial to success in a nursing program. The section is divided into three main areas:

1. **Key Ideas and Details**: Involving 22 questions, this section probes into your ability to summarize texts, make logical inferences, understand sequences of events, and locate specific details. You'll encounter charts, graphs, and other visual data and be asked to interpret and apply the provided information.
2. **Craft and Structure**: Consisting of 14 questions, this section tests your skills in differentiating between fact and opinion, using context to define words, evaluating the author's purpose and viewpoint, and understanding the organization of texts.
3. **Integration of Knowledge and Ideas**: This part, made up of 11 questions, demands the skill to make predictions and draw conclusions using evidence from the text, compare themes, and evaluate arguments. It will also require you to integrate data from multiple sources.

In addition, there are 6 pretest questions that are not scored.

The texts provided can range from simple, straightforward passages to more complex, multi-paragraph texts. The ability to understand and make use of written information is an integral part of healthcare delivery, and this section is designed to ensure you possess these critical skills. The diverse types of questions will challenge your ability to actively engage with a text, analyze it, and apply its information to different scenarios. Thus, performing well in this section sets a solid foundation for success in your future nursing career.

Key Ideas and Details:

Understanding and summarizing texts is crucial in the field of nursing. In this profession, you're frequently exposed to a multitude of information, including patient records, research studies, and procedural manuals. These documents are often laden with crucial details that need to be understood and communicated effectively to ensure patient safety and proper care.

Summarizing is a skill that allows you to distill complex texts into a concise explanation that retains the key points. By summarizing, you are essentially processing the information and making it easier to understand and recall. This practice promotes your understanding of the material, aids in retaining information, and improves your ability to communicate these details to others.

For instance, summarizing a patient's case history can help you recall crucial details about their condition and treatment plan. This could lead to better care decisions and more effective communication with other healthcare professionals. Similarly, summarizing the findings of a recent medical study could help you understand its implications for your practice and communicate this to colleagues or patients.

In summary, the ability to understand and summarize text not only aids reading comprehension but also enhances your ability to make informed decisions and communicate effectively, both of which are essential skills in nursing.

Crafting an effective summary requires a keen understanding of the text and the ability to extract and present the most significant information in a succinct manner. Here are some strategies to help you achieve this:
1. **Read the entire text first:** Before attempting to summarize, ensure you've read the full text to grasp its overall meaning and context. This holistic understanding forms the backbone of your summary.
2. **Identify the main idea:** Each passage typically has a central theme or main idea. This is often found in the introduction or conclusion but can be embedded throughout the text. Identifying the main idea is crucial for preserving the essence of the text in your summary.
3. **Highlight key points:** While reading, mark or note significant points, arguments, or pieces of evidence that support the main idea. This can help you remember and extract key elements for your summary.
4. **Condense information:** Remove any superfluous details, examples, or repetitive information. Aim to simplify complex phrases and sentences without altering their original meaning.
5. **Use your own words:** Paraphrase the author's ideas into your own words. This encourages active understanding and helps to ensure that the summary is in your voice.
6. **Check your work:** Finally, review your summary to ensure it accurately represents the main idea and key points from the original text. Ask yourself: "If someone read my summary, would they grasp the main idea and essential elements of the text?"

Remember, a summary should be a distilled version of the text that remains true to the original content. The goal is not just to shorten the text, but to present the key information in a clear, concise manner.

Inference and conclusion drawing play pivotal roles in reading comprehension, allowing us to uncover meaning not explicitly stated in the text. This nuanced understanding deepens our engagement with the material, enhances critical thinking, and empowers us to extrapolate information useful in various contexts.

Consider inference as connecting the dots. As readers, we gather information provided by the author and combine it with our prior knowledge and experiences. This amalgamation enables us to fill gaps, predict outcomes, and grasp implicit meanings. For instance, if a passage describes a character shivering with a runny nose, we might infer they are cold or ill, even if it's not expressly stated.

As for drawing conclusions, it's the process of making a judgement or decision based on the information at hand. For instance, after reading a piece about climate change with various data on rising global temperatures, a reader might conclude that immediate actions are necessary to mitigate these changes.

Improving these skills requires deliberate practice and can be enhanced with the following strategies:

1. **Read actively:** Engage with the text, questioning it and making predictions. This encourages mental interaction with the material, facilitating inferential reasoning and conclusion drawing.
2. **Note context clues:** Pay attention to the author's language, tone, and style. Words and phrases surrounding an idea can give hints about its meaning.
3. **Use prior knowledge:** Connect the new information with what you already know. This can help to interpret indirect information and make educated guesses.
4. **Practice with diverse texts:** Different genres and styles of text require various inference skills. Regularly reading a broad range of materials can help to strengthen these abilities.
5. **Discuss and reflect:** Discuss your interpretations with peers or mentors. This can expose you to different perspectives and reinforce your understanding. Reflect on the reading process and the strategies you've used to infer and conclude.

Remember, these skills aren't just for reading comprehension. They're tools for critical thinking that you'll use throughout your nursing career and daily life. So, be patient with yourself and celebrate each small improvement. You're not just studying for an exam; you're building a foundation for a successful future.

The ability to interpret written directions and decipher graphs and charts is an integral skill in a healthcare setting. From medication instructions and patient charts to diagnostic reports and research data, these elements form the backbone of effective communication and informed decision-making in healthcare.

Here are some strategies to enhance these skills:

1. **Active Reading:** Approach written instructions or data with an active mind, aiming to understand the underlying meaning rather than simply reading the words.
2. **Break It Down:** If instructions are lengthy or complex, break them down into smaller, manageable parts. Understand each step before moving on to the next.
3. **Identify Key Information:** For graphs and charts, pay attention to titles, labels, axes, and legends. These contain vital information that will guide your interpretation.
4. **Analyze Trends:** Look for patterns or trends in the data. In graphs, pay attention to the direction (increasing or decreasing) and speed of change.
5. **Verify Understanding:** After interpreting, ensure your understanding aligns with the data or instructions given. You might want to summarize or explain it to another person.

In healthcare, misinterpreting instructions can have serious consequences. For instance, consider a nurse administering medication. Accurate interpretation of the written dosage instructions is crucial. A misunderstanding could lead to administering the wrong dose, risking the patient's health.

Similarly, a healthcare provider might need to interpret a patient's blood glucose levels chart to assess diabetes management. Misinterpreting the data trends could lead to inappropriate treatment recommendations.

Interpreting graphs and charts is also important in staying informed about recent research or understanding public health information. For example, during a viral outbreak, healthcare professionals need to understand charts tracking infection rates, recovery rates, and mortality rates to make informed decisions about treatment strategies and patient advice.

Remember, practice makes perfect. Regularly engage with different types of written instructions, graphs, and charts to become more comfortable and proficient with them. This isn't just a skill for your TEAS exam; it's a lifelong tool for your nursing career.

Craft and Structure:

Being able to differentiate between fact and opinion is a skill of paramount importance in healthcare, particularly in the nursing profession. It's essential in providing evidence-based care, promoting informed patient decision-making, and interacting professionally with colleagues.

Let's begin with the basics. A fact is a statement that can be proven true or false. It's objective and verifiable. An opinion, on the other hand, is a subjective statement based on beliefs or personal views. It cannot be conclusively proven or disproven.

In the nursing field, the ability to discern facts from opinions is particularly important for several reasons:

1. **Evidence-Based Practice:** Nurses rely on facts (evidence) to guide their clinical decisions. Misinterpreting an opinion as fact could lead to ineffective or harmful care. For instance, a factual statement would be: "Studies show that regular physical activity can help manage type 2 diabetes." An opinion might be: "I think yoga is the best type of exercise for individuals with diabetes."
2. **Patient Education:** When educating patients about their health or treatment options, it's vital to communicate factual information to support informed decision-making. Personal opinions should be clearly marked as such, to avoid confusion.
3. **Professional Communication:** Nurses must effectively communicate with a diverse healthcare team. Using facts to support statements ensures accuracy and clarity. For example, saying "The patient's blood pressure has been consistently above 140/90 mmHg today" is factual and provides clear information for decision-making.

So, how can a nurse refine the skill of distinguishing facts from opinions? Here are a few strategies:

- **Critical Thinking:** Evaluate the statement. Can it be proven true or false? Is there empirical evidence to support it, or is it based on personal beliefs or feelings?
- **Source Evaluation:** Consider the source of the information. Scientific studies, official health department reports, and medical guidelines usually offer factual information. Personal blogs, social media, and casual conversations may contain more opinion-based content.

- **Asking Questions:** When in doubt, ask questions. Seek clarification and ask for the evidence supporting the statement.

Understanding the distinction between facts and opinions is not only crucial for your TEAS exam but also for your future nursing career. It underpins effective, ethical, and patient-centered care.

Context clues are essential tools for deciphering unfamiliar words or phrases in a text. They can be found within the same sentence or in surrounding sentences, and they offer hints about a word's meaning. The ability to use context clues is particularly valuable when reading technical or medical texts, where specialized terminology is common.

Let's explore four types of context clues and strategies for using them:

1. **Definition Clues:** The text directly provides the meaning of an unfamiliar term. A colon, comma, or the word 'is' often introduces the definition. For example, in the sentence "Hypertension, a condition characterized by consistently high blood pressure, is common in adults," 'a condition characterized by consistently high blood pressure' is the definition of 'hypertension.'
2. **Synonym Clues:** The text includes a synonym or similar word to the unfamiliar term. An example could be, "The doctor prescribed an analgesic, a painkiller, to help manage her symptoms." Here, 'painkiller' is a synonym for 'analgesic.'
3. **Antonym Clues:** The text offers an antonym or contrast to the unfamiliar word. Words like 'but,' 'however,' or 'unlike' often signal antonym clues. For example, "Unlike benign tumors, malignant tumors can invade nearby tissues and spread to other parts of the body." Here, 'benign' is contrasted with 'malignant.'
4. **Example Clues:** The text provides examples to help understand the unfamiliar term. Words such as 'including,' 'for example,' or 'such as' often introduce these clues. An example sentence could be, "The nurse used several aseptic techniques, such as hand washing and using sterilized equipment."

Understanding context clues can dramatically improve comprehension and fluency, especially in complex medical texts. Here are some strategies to enhance this skill:

- **Read Around the Word:** Don't focus only on the unfamiliar term. Look at the surrounding text for potential clues about its meaning.
- **Practice:** Regularly reading technical and medical texts can help develop this skill. Try to infer the meaning of unfamiliar words before looking them up, then check your understanding.
- **Identify Clue Types:** Familiarize yourself with different types of context clues and look out for words or punctuation that often signal them.
- **Use a Dictionary:** After using context clues, confirm your inference using a dictionary. This also helps expand your vocabulary.

By mastering the use of context clues, you'll be well equipped not only to tackle the TEAS exam but also to navigate the dense medical literature you'll encounter in your nursing career.

When you evaluate an author's purpose and point of view, you're delving into the reasons behind their creation of the text and the perspective from which they're approaching the topic.

This examination allows you to go beyond the surface-level understanding of the text and navigate the nuances, potential biases, and underlying messages embedded within it. This skill is fundamental in enhancing critical reading, a vital attribute for any aspiring nurse, as it leads to better comprehension and interpretation of a variety of documents, from medical studies to patient narratives.

Authors typically write for one of three main purposes: to inform, to persuade, or to entertain. Sometimes, they may aim to achieve a combination of these. By discerning the author's primary purpose, you can better interpret the text and align your reading approach to suit it.

Point of view, on the other hand, pertains to the author's position or attitude towards the topic at hand. It's through this lens that the information is presented, and understanding it can offer you a more profound comprehension of the text.

Let's consider a couple of examples:

1. Suppose you're reading an article advocating for a new vaccination strategy. The author's purpose may be to persuade the reader about the effectiveness of this strategy. Their point of view may be positive towards the strategy due to their belief in its potential benefits. Understanding this can guide you in critically assessing the arguments presented, perhaps prompting you to look for other sources to compare different perspectives and ensure a balanced understanding.
2. If you're perusing a research paper about a medical trial's results, the author's purpose is likely to inform. They may present the data neutrally, but their point of view could become apparent in how they interpret the data or suggest implications for future practice. Understanding their perspective can help you scrutinize the interpretations and conclusions drawn.

In summary, evaluating an author's purpose and point of view is a fundamental reading skill that deepens your understanding of the text and promotes critical thinking—a crucial ability in the nursing field. Not only does it prepare you for the TEAS exam, but it also equips you for comprehending a wide array of professional resources in your future career.

Integration of Knowledge and Ideas:

The process of integrating knowledge and ideas from various sources entails gathering, comparing, analyzing, and synthesizing information from a range of resources to form a comprehensive understanding of a topic. It's about looking at the "bigger picture," piecing together different perspectives, facts, and theories to form a holistic view.

In a healthcare setting, this ability is indispensable. Here's why:

1. Diverse Information Sources: Healthcare professionals regularly interact with a plethora of information, from medical research papers and clinical guidelines to patient histories and consultation notes. Each of these sources presents a piece of the puzzle, and by integrating this information, healthcare providers can make more informed, accurate decisions.
2. Interdisciplinary Nature: Healthcare is innately interdisciplinary, requiring knowledge from various fields such as biology, pharmacology, psychology, sociology, and more. The

ability to integrate ideas across these disciplines enables a more comprehensive approach to patient care.
3. Enhancing Patient Care: A healthcare professional's primary goal is to deliver effective, personalized patient care. By integrating knowledge from different sources - like patient symptoms, lab results, clinical research, and even a patient's social situation - they can devise a care plan that addresses the patient's unique needs and circumstances.
4. Continual Learning: The healthcare field is continuously evolving with new research findings, treatment methodologies, and technological advancements. Professionals must constantly integrate new knowledge into their existing understanding to stay current and provide the best possible care.

Take, for example, a nurse working with a patient who has been diagnosed with a chronic disease. The nurse would need to integrate information from the patient's medical history, current symptoms, research on the disease, pharmacological data on prescribed drugs, and perhaps even the patient's lifestyle and emotional state to provide comprehensive care.

So, integrating knowledge and ideas isn't just a skill required for the TEAS—it's a fundamental aspect of nursing practice. It supports evidence-based decision-making, patient-centered care, and the continual learning that is vital in the rapidly evolving field of healthcare.

Developing the ability to integrate information from various sources is akin to becoming a detective. You're piecing together a comprehensive and accurate picture of a subject from multiple perspectives. Here are a few strategies to help you with this process:
1. Source Identification: Recognize the different sources available to you, both primary and secondary. Primary sources come straight from the source, such as patient histories in healthcare. Secondary sources interpret or analyze primary sources, such as a review of clinical trials.
2. Cross-Referencing: Look for commonalities and differences in the information provided by different sources. When multiple reliable sources agree on a piece of information, it's more likely to be accurate.
3. Critical Analysis: Don't take everything at face value. Consider the purpose and context of the information, and critically analyze its relevance and reliability.
4. Synthesize Information: After gathering and evaluating information, draw together your conclusions to form a cohesive understanding of the topic. This could involve noting patterns, identifying key themes, or relating new knowledge to what you already know.
5. Organize Your Thoughts: Use tools like outlines, diagrams, or mind maps to help visualize and arrange the information you're integrating.

To verify the accuracy and reliability of information, especially from secondary sources, consider the following:
1. Source Credibility: Who is the author, and what are their qualifications? Is the source reputable?
2. Purpose of the Information: Why was the information published? Is it intended to inform, persuade, or sell something?

3. Evidence-Based: Is the information backed up by evidence? In the context of healthcare, this would typically mean clinical research, case studies, or verified medical statistics.
4. Date of Publication: Is the information up-to-date? In fields like medicine, where new discoveries are continuously being made, this is particularly important.
5. Consistency: Does the information agree with what's provided by other credible sources?

By applying these strategies, you can efficiently integrate information from various sources while ensuring its accuracy and reliability.

The integration of knowledge and ideas is like putting together the pieces of a complex puzzle. In nursing practice, this skill is crucial as it involves multiple data sources to form a holistic understanding of a patient's health status and develop a tailored care plan.

Consider this scenario: A patient comes in with a persistent cough and fatigue. A newly-graduated nurse might immediately think of a common cold. However, an experienced nurse knows to integrate knowledge from different areas. They consider the patient's age, lifestyle, recent travels, family history, and the prevalence of certain diseases in their community. They don't just look at the immediate symptoms; they also consider lab reports, chest X-rays, and possibly even environmental factors.

Suppose the patient is a smoker, has a family history of lung cancer, and the chest X-ray reveals a mass in the lung. The nurse can't diagnose, but these pieces of information raise suspicion of a more serious condition like lung cancer. Here, the nurse used the integration of knowledge and ideas from different sources, including the patient's history, current symptoms, diagnostic tests, and knowledge of risk factors for various diseases.

In another scenario, a nurse might be caring for a patient with diabetes. They'll need to integrate knowledge from nutrition (to advise on diet), pharmacology (to manage insulin), and psychology (to motivate lifestyle changes), along with the patient's personal preferences and cultural beliefs. Only with this integrated approach can they develop a truly effective care plan.

By pulling together varied strands of information, nurses can get a fuller picture of their patients' health and make better-informed decisions about their care. This skill of integration leads to improved patient outcomes, better resource allocation, and increased efficiency in healthcare delivery.

MATHEMATICS SECTION:

Delving into the Mathematics section of the ATI TEAS Exam (7th Edition), it's important to note that it primarily gauges the quantitative skills essential in a healthcare context, especially nursing. This section comprises 36 questions, each carefully designed to assess your ability to reason, solve problems, and interpret data using mathematical concepts.

Here's a broad overview of the subtopics we will cover in this section:

1. **Numbers and Algebra:** This section primarily concerns numerical operations, including addition, subtraction, multiplication, and division. It further delves into algebraic equations and the use of integers, fractions, ratios, proportions, and percentages. Our focus will be on practical applications, particularly as they relate to healthcare scenarios.
2. **Measurement and Data:** This subsection is all about measurement units and conversions. You'll learn to interpret various forms of data presentation such as tables, graphs, charts, and diagrams. We'll also cover probability and statistics as they relate to healthcare, like understanding patient data.

Throughout the Mathematics chapter, our goal will be to impart not only an understanding of basic mathematical operations and concepts but also the ability to apply this knowledge to real-world healthcare scenarios. By the end of this chapter, you should feel confident in performing basic mathematical operations, interpreting data, and solving problems relevant to a healthcare setting.

Get ready to tackle the Mathematics section with focus and determination! With practice and understanding, you will master these concepts and enhance your quantitative reasoning skills, essential tools for your future nursing practice.

Rational numbers are numbers that can be expressed as the quotient, or a fraction, of two integers, where the denominator is not zero. In other words, if you have a number that can be written as a/b where a and b are integers, and b is not zero, then you have a rational number.

Examples of rational numbers include simple fractions like 1/2, 2/3, whole numbers (which can be expressed as the number over 1, like 4/1), and numbers with finite or repeating decimal points, like 0.5 (which is 1/2) or 0.333... (which is 1/3).

Integers, on the other hand, are a subset of rational numbers. They include whole numbers and their negatives, but not fractions or decimals. For example, -2, -1, 0, 1, 2 are all integers.

In a healthcare setting, rational numbers are quite ubiquitous. They come up in dosages of medication, in nutritional information, in the reading of various instruments, and in the interpretation of various medical tests. For instance, a doctor may prescribe a 0.5mg tablet of a certain medication, a nurse might administer 2/3 of an IV bag, or a dietitian might recommend that a patient gets 1/3 of their calories from carbohydrates. In each of these examples, we are dealing with rational numbers.

Understanding the concept of rational numbers is thus crucial for healthcare professionals, as accurate calculations can significantly affect patient care and outcomes. Misunderstanding or miscalculating a dosage or proportion can have serious consequences. Therefore, mastering rational numbers is not just part of passing your exam but an integral skill for your future nursing career.

let's look at **how to solve both simple and complex equations.**
1. **Simple Equation**

A simple equation might look something like this:

x + 7 = 12

The goal here is to solve for **x**. We can do this by subtracting **7** from both sides of the equation:

x + 7 - 7 = 12 - 7

This simplifies to:

x = 5

And that's it. In this equation, **x** equals **5**.

2. **Complex Equation**

Now, let's look at a more complex equation that might involve multiple operations. For example:

3x - 7 = 20

The goal here is still to solve for **x**. We can begin by adding **7** to both sides of the equation to isolate the term with **x**:

3x - 7 + 7 = 20 + 7

Which simplifies to:

3x = 27

Next, to solve for **x**, we divide both sides by **3**:

3x / 3 = 27 / 3

And this simplifies to:

x = 9

So in this case, **x** equals **9**.

Remember that the same principles apply regardless of the complexity of the equation. Your goal is to isolate the variable by using inverse operations (addition/subtraction, multiplication/division) on both sides of the equation to maintain equality.

It's also worth noting that in nursing, these skills are very important, especially when calculating medication dosages, interpreting data, and solving problems related to patient care. The TEAS math section ensures you have these basic algebraic skills to succeed in your nursing program and future career.

Algebraic equations have an essential place in nursing. They are the foundation of many daily tasks and considerations that healthcare professionals must manage. Here are a few examples:
1. **Medication Dosage Calculations**: Nurses often need to determine the correct medication dosage for a patient. Dosages might be based on a patient's weight or other variables. For instance, if a medication dose is prescribed as 5 mg per kg of body weight,

a nurse would use an algebraic equation to calculate the precise dosage for a patient's specific weight.
2. **Drip Rates**: When administering intravenous (IV) medications, nurses need to calculate the drip rate (drops per minute), which often involves solving an algebraic equation. The formula typically includes the volume of the fluid, the drop factor of the IV tubing, and the desired time frame.
3. **Concentration Problems**: Sometimes, a nurse may need to dilute a medication or solution to a particular concentration. Algebra can help determine the amount of solute and solvent needed to achieve the desired concentration.
4. **Body Mass Index (BMI)**: BMI is calculated using an individual's weight and height. Nurses often calculate BMI to determine if a patient's weight is in a healthy range.
5. **Nutritional Needs**: Certain nutritional needs, such as caloric intake or fluid requirements, can be calculated using algebraic equations, considering factors like the patient's weight, age, and health status.
6. **Health Metrics**: Various health metrics, such as creatinine clearance or estimated glomerular filtration rate (eGFR), require algebra to calculate. These measures are crucial for assessing kidney function.

These are just a few examples, but they highlight the vital role that algebraic equations play in nursing. Being comfortable with algebra can ensure accuracy, promote patient safety, and enhance overall patient care.

Working with Rational Numbers:

Rational numbers are a category of numbers that includes integers, fractions, and decimal numbers that terminate or repeat. Essentially, a rational number can be expressed as a fraction where both the numerator (top number) and the denominator (bottom number) are integers, and the denominator is not zero.

For instance, consider the numbers 5, -3, 1/2, and 0.75.
- 5 is a rational number because it can be expressed as 5/1.
- -3 is a rational number as it can be expressed as -3/1.
- 1/2 is a rational number because it's already expressed as a fraction with integer values in the numerator and the denominator.
- 0.75 is a rational number as it can be written as the fraction 3/4.

Rational numbers are everywhere in healthcare. They could represent the dosage of medication to administer (e.g., 0.5 mg of a drug), the rate of an intravenous drip (like 60 drops per minute, which could be seen as a ratio of 60:1), or a patient's body mass index (a ratio of weight to height squared). Understanding and working with rational numbers is thus critical in the healthcare setting.

Solving Equations:

Performing basic operations with rational numbers, particularly fractions, requires understanding a few foundational steps. Let's break down each operation:
1. **Addition/Subtraction:** When adding or subtracting rational numbers (expressed as fractions), they must have the same denominator (known as a common denominator). If they don't, you'll have to find equivalent fractions that do.

For instance, to add 1/4 and 2/3, first find a common denominator. The least common denominator for 4 and 3 is 12. Convert each fraction to have this denominator: 1/4 becomes 3/12 and 2/3 becomes 8/12. Now, add the numerators: 3 + 8 = 11. So, 1/4 + 2/3 = 11/12.

2. **Multiplication:** Multiplication is simpler than addition or subtraction. You simply multiply the numerators together to form the new numerator, and multiply the denominators to form the new denominator.

For example, to multiply 3/4 by 2/5, multiply the numerators (3*2 = 6) and the denominators (4*5 = 20), to get 6/20. Simplify the result, if possible, to get 3/10.

3. **Division:** When dividing fractions, you multiply the first fraction by the reciprocal of the second.

Let's say we're dividing 3/4 by 2/5. The reciprocal of 2/5 is 5/2. So, you'd multiply 3/4 by 5/2. Following the multiplication rule we just discussed, you'd get (3*5)/(4*2) = 15/8.

Note: When dealing with decimals, operations are handled similarly to whole numbers. However, take care with place values when adding, subtracting, and multiplying decimals. For division, you may need to move the decimal point in the divisor (the number you're dividing by) to make it a whole number, doing the same operation to the dividend (the number being divided).

In every case, when dealing with negative rational numbers, remember that two negatives make a positive (for multiplication and division), and subtracting a negative is equivalent to adding a positive.

Solving algebraic equations can sometimes be a tricky task, but there are several effective strategies you can employ to make the process simpler:
1. **Understand the Order of Operations:** This is a basic rule that you must follow while solving equations. The order is usually remembered by the acronym PEMDAS (Parentheses, Exponents, Multiplication and Division (from left to right), Addition and Subtraction (from left to right)).
2. **Combining Like Terms:** This involves simplifying the equation by adding or subtracting similar terms. For example, in the equation 3x + 5 - 2x = 12, you can combine '3x' and '-2x' to simplify the equation to 'x + 5 = 12'.
3. **Applying the Addition/Subtraction Property of Equality:** If you add or subtract the same number from both sides of the equation, it keeps the equation balanced. For example, using the simplified equation 'x + 5 = 12', you can subtract 5 from both sides to isolate x, giving you 'x = 7'.

4. **Applying the Multiplication/Division Property of Equality:** Similar to the addition/subtraction property, if you multiply or divide both sides of the equation by the same nonzero number, the equation stays balanced. For example, if you have the equation '2x = 8', you can divide both sides by 2 to solve for x, giving 'x = 4'.
5. **Checking Your Answer:** Once you've solved the equation, it's always a good idea to check your work. Substitute the value of the variable back into the original equation to ensure both sides remain equal.
6. **Breaking Down Complex Equations:** If you're working with a more complex equation, try to break it down into simpler parts. Look for opportunities to factor or to simplify complex fractions.

By using these strategies consistently and with practice, your skills at solving algebraic equations should improve significantly.

let's explore a few types of algebraic equations and how to solve them:
1. **Linear Equation:** This is the simplest type of equation, where the highest power of the variable is 1. For example, $3x + 2 = 8$. You can solve it by first subtracting 2 from both sides, giving $3x = 6$, and then dividing both sides by 3, resulting in $x = 2$.
2. **Quadratic Equation:** This type of equation includes a term with a variable raised to the second power. For example, $x^2 - 5x + 6 = 0$. This quadratic can be factored into $(x - 2)(x - 3) = 0$, which yields solutions of $x = 2$ and $x = 3$.
3. **Equation with Fractions (Rational Equations):** Sometimes, variables occur in the denominator of a fraction. For example, $1/(x - 2) + 1/(x - 3) = 1$. To solve this, you would find a common denominator, combine terms, and then cross-multiply to solve for x.
4. **Radical Equation:** These equations involve roots, such as square roots. For instance, $\sqrt{(x - 2)} = 3$. To solve this, you would first square both sides to get rid of the square root, resulting in $x - 2 = 9$. Then, add 2 to both sides to solve for x, yielding $x = 11$.
5. **Exponential Equation:** Here, the variable is in the exponent, such as $2^x = 8$. To solve this, you can write both sides with the same base (since 8 is 2^3), resulting in $2^x = 2^3$. Therefore, x must equal 3.

These examples represent a few types of algebraic equations you might encounter. The steps to solve them can vary greatly depending on the complexity and form of the equation.

Real-world Problem Solving (Percentages, Proportions, Ratios, etc.):

percentages, proportions, and ratios are fundamental to nursing practice in a variety of ways. Let's delve into each one and see how they're applied:
1. **Percentages:** Percentages are used in a myriad of ways in nursing. For instance, nurses often need to calculate the percentage of weight loss or gain in patients. This requires taking the difference in weight and dividing it by the original weight, then multiplying by 100 to convert to a percentage. Another common usage is in calculating body surface area (BSA) for medication dosage, where percentages are used to estimate the body's surface area for appropriate drug dosing.

2. **Proportions**: Proportions are especially useful in the context of medication dosages. For instance, if a medication is to be delivered at a specific rate, say 5 mg per kg of body weight, a nurse would need to proportionally adjust the dosage based on the patient's actual weight. If a child weighs 20 kg, the dosage would be proportionally adjusted to 100 mg (5 mg/kg x 20 kg = 100 mg).
3. **Ratios**: Ratios are prevalent in many nursing scenarios, such as determining the concentration of a solution, or the proportion of one component to another. For example, intravenous (IV) solutions may be mixed in certain ratios, like a 1:10 ratio means one part of the drug to ten parts of the diluent. Nurses also use ratios in the calculation of heart and respiratory rates, where they compare the number of breaths or heartbeats to time.

These mathematical concepts are not just abstract ideas but have real-life, practical implications in the healthcare field, particularly in nursing. They assist in ensuring accurate measurements, precise medication dosages, and effective monitoring, all of which contribute significantly to patient care and safety.

Solving problems involving percentages, proportions, and ratios involves a series of steps and some helpful strategies. Here's a broad approach for each:

1. **Percentages**: When dealing with percentages, it's crucial to remember that 'percent' means 'per 100'. So, when you see 50%, think '50 per 100', or 0.5 when expressed as a decimal. One strategy is to convert percentages to decimals or fractions before performing calculations. For example, to calculate 20% of 50, you can convert 20% to 0.2, then multiply by 50 to get the answer.
2. **Proportions**: A proportion is an equation that states two ratios are equal. To solve problems involving proportions, use the cross-multiplication method. For example, if $a/b = c/d$ and you know the values of a, b, and c but not d, you can solve for d by cross-multiplying: $ad = bc$. Then, solve for d by dividing both sides by a.
3. **Ratios**: When working with ratios, remember that they represent a relationship between two quantities. If you're given a ratio of 4:5 and asked to find out what number corresponds to 5 when 4 corresponds to 20, you can set up a proportion (4/20 = 5/x), and solve for x using cross-multiplication.

When solving these types of problems, always check your answer to ensure it makes sense in the context of the original problem. Practice is crucial in becoming proficient at solving problems with percentages, proportions, and ratios. With time, these methods will become second nature.

Measurement and Data:

Data interpretation is an essential skill in healthcare settings. It involves gathering, analyzing, and making conclusions based on a variety of data sources. Here are a few ways data interpretation is used in healthcare:

1. **Patient Care**: Healthcare professionals regularly review and interpret data like lab results, vital signs, patient symptoms, and more to make informed decisions about patient care. For example, a nurse may need to interpret blood pressure readings over time to determine if a patient's medication regimen is effective.
2. **Research**: Healthcare research often involves interpreting statistical data to draw conclusions about health outcomes, efficacy of treatments, or disease prevalence. For instance, analyzing data from a clinical trial could lead to the discovery of a new, more effective treatment regimen for a particular disease.
3. **Quality Improvement**: Healthcare facilities often collect and analyze data related to patient outcomes, satisfaction scores, and operational efficiency. Interpreting this data can lead to improvements in the care patients receive. For example, analysis of patient satisfaction surveys can provide insights into areas where a healthcare facility is performing well and where improvements can be made.
4. **Public Health**: In public health, data interpretation can inform strategies to address health issues at a population level. For instance, analyzing epidemiological data during a disease outbreak can help identify patterns of transmission and inform interventions.

In each of these examples, the ability to accurately interpret data directly impacts the quality of care provided and health outcomes. It's important for healthcare professionals to develop strong data interpretation skills to support their decision-making process.

Interpreting Data from Tables and Charts:

Interpreting data from tables, charts, and graphs involves a number of steps:
1. **Identify the Type of Display**: Start by figuring out whether you're looking at a table, bar graph, line graph, pie chart, or another type of display. Different displays are better suited to different types of data, so identifying the format can provide hints about what the data represents.
2. **Read the Title and Labels**: The title should give you a good idea of what the data represents, while the labels will define the different data points or categories. If there's a legend, make sure to understand what each symbol or color represents.
3. **Identify the Variables**: Understand what each axis in a graph or column in a table represents. In most graphs, the x-axis (horizontal) represents the independent variable and the y-axis (vertical) represents the dependent variable.
4. **Examine the Scale**: Check the scales on the axes in a graph. Are they linear, logarithmic, or something else? A glance might not reveal the true nature of the data if the scales are not understood correctly.
5. **Analyze the Data**: Look for patterns, trends, or anomalies in the data. In a line graph, for instance, you might look for an overall upward or downward trend. In a bar graph, you might compare the lengths of the bars.
6. **Draw Conclusions**: Based on your analysis, what can you infer from the data? Do the data points suggest a particular conclusion or trend?

7. **Consider the Source and Methodology**: Remember to consider where the data came from. Is it likely to be reliable and unbiased? Were there any limitations in how the data was collected that might impact your interpretation?

By using these steps as a guide, you can navigate different types of data displays with greater confidence and accuracy.

here are some examples of how interpreting data from tables and charts might look in a healthcare context:

1. **Patient's Vitals Over Time**: Let's say you're presented with a chart displaying a patient's heart rate over a 24-hour period. The Y-axis represents heart rate (beats per minute), and the X-axis represents time. Seeing a general trend of stability with minor fluctuations would be expected. However, if you notice dramatic spikes or dips, it may indicate a medical event that needs attention.
2. **Medication Dosage**: You might be given a table that represents the various dosages of medication a patient has taken over several days, with the date in the first column and the type and amount of medication in the subsequent columns. Consistency in the administration of the drug would be a positive sign, while inconsistencies could indicate potential problems with the treatment plan.
3. **Lab Results**: Another example could be a chart displaying lab results, such as blood glucose levels. This would typically be a line chart with time on the X-axis and glucose concentration on the Y-axis. Consistent readings within the normal range would be ideal, whereas values that fall outside the normal range or show large fluctuations might signal a need for further investigation or intervention.
4. **Epidemiological Data**: You might need to interpret a bar graph illustrating the incidence of a particular disease over time in different populations. This type of data is crucial for understanding the spread of diseases and planning public health interventions.

These examples illustrate how critical the ability to interpret tables and charts can be in the healthcare field. This skill can quite literally be a lifesaver, allowing healthcare providers to monitor patient health, track the progression of illnesses, and evaluate the effectiveness of treatments.

Calculating Geometric Quantities:

understanding geometric quantities can be quite pertinent in the nursing field, and here are some examples to illustrate this:

1. **Wound Care**: If you're assessing a patient's wound, you'll need to estimate its size to monitor healing progress and plan for treatment. You may need to approximate the wound's length, width, and sometimes even depth - all of which involve concepts of geometry.
2. **Dosage Calculations**: Certain medications are dosed based on the patient's body surface area, particularly in chemotherapy. The calculation of body surface area is a geometric concept, as it involves understanding two-dimensional measurements.

3. **Medical Imaging**: Nurses often work with radiologists or other medical imaging specialists, where geometric principles come into play. For instance, understanding angles and projections can help in positioning the patient correctly for an x-ray or a scan.
4. **Assisting in Procedures**: Nurses may need to assist in procedures that require a knowledge of geometry. For example, during the insertion of an IV, understanding angles can be helpful to ensure the correct insertion angle is used.
5. **Mobility Assessment**: Assessing a patient's range of motion in their joints is another practical application of geometry. Using the concept of angles, you can measure the extent of a patient's mobility or flexibility.

In all these scenarios, a nurse's knowledge of geometric quantities isn't just academic; it has very real and practical implications for patient care. By understanding these concepts, a nurse can make accurate assessments, administer the appropriate treatments, and monitor a patient's progress effectively.

Being able to calculate geometric quantities such as areas and volumes can be quite handy. Below, you'll find tips for calculating these quantities in common shapes:

1. **Area of a rectangle**: The area of a rectangle is found by multiplying the length by the width (Area = length x width). So, if you have a rectangle that is 4 units long and 3 units wide, the area would be 4 units x 3 units = 12 square units.
2. **Area of a triangle**: The area of a triangle is found by multiplying the base by the height and then dividing by 2 (Area = 1/2 base x height). So, if a triangle has a base of 5 units and a height of 6 units, the area would be (1/2) x 5 units x 6 units = 15 square units.
3. **Area of a circle**: The area of a circle is found using the formula Area = πr^2 (where r is the radius). Thus, if you have a circle with a radius of 3 units, the area would be π x (3 units)^2 = 9π square units.
4. **Volume of a rectangular prism (box)**: The volume of a rectangular prism is found by multiplying the length by the width and the height (Volume = length x width x height). If a box is 2 units long, 3 units wide, and 4 units high, the volume would be 2 units x 3 units x 4 units = 24 cubic units.
5. **Volume of a cylinder**: The volume of a cylinder is found using the formula Volume = $\pi r^2 h$ (where r is the radius of the base circle and h is the height). If a cylinder has a radius of 3 units and a height of 5 units, the volume would be π x (3 units)^2 x 5 units = 45π cubic units.
6. **Volume of a sphere**: The volume of a sphere is given by the formula Volume = $4/3 \pi r^3$ (where r is the radius). So, if a sphere has a radius of 2 units, the volume would be $4/3\pi$ x (2 units)^3 = $32/3\pi$ cubic units.

Remember, these are simple formulas to keep in mind, but actual problem-solving may require understanding and application of these principles in a step-by-step manner. Practicing these calculations will help you become more comfortable with them over time.

Unit Conversion:

Unit conversion is indeed crucial in nursing, primarily because healthcare is an international endeavor that uses a variety of measurement systems. Inaccurate conversions can lead to serious medical errors, sometimes even life-threatening ones. Here are some instances where unit conversion plays a significant role in a healthcare setting:
1. **Medication Dosages**: Medication dosages are usually prescribed in a specific unit of measurement, like milligrams (mg) or micrograms (mcg). Nurses often need to convert these units based on the form and concentration of the medication available. For example, a doctor might prescribe a medication dosage of 500mg, but the medication on hand might be in a solution of 250mg/5ml. The nurse would need to convert the prescribed dosage into a volume (ml) for accurate administration.
2. **Patient Weight and Height**: The patient's weight and height can impact the dosage of medication required. These are often measured in kilograms (kg) and centimeters (cm) in most countries. However, in the United States, these measurements are often taken in pounds (lbs) and inches (in). Nurses need to be able to convert these units to ensure accurate medication dosing.
3. **IV Drip Rates**: Intravenous (IV) medications may need to be administered at a particular rate. This rate might be prescribed in ml/hour, but the nurse might need to set the drip rate on the IV pump in drops/minute, based on the specific type of tubing used. Correct conversions between these units are essential to maintain the correct medication dosage.
4. **Laboratory Results**: Lab results can come in a variety of units, which might need to be converted to interpret the results accurately and to compare with standard or desired ranges. For example, glucose levels might be reported in mmol/L, but some practitioners might be more accustomed to mg/dL.

These examples illustrate why competency in unit conversions is a fundamental skill in nursing. An incorrect conversion could lead to a significant medical error, so it's essential to understand and accurately carry out these conversions to ensure patient safety.

Let's discuss some common unit conversions you might encounter in a healthcare setting.
Example 1: Converting Patient Weight from Pounds (lbs) to Kilograms (kg)
Healthcare providers often measure patient weight in pounds, especially in the United States, but many medical calculations require weight in kilograms.
Let's say a patient weighs 150 lbs. To convert this to kilograms, we use the conversion factor 1 kg = 2.20462 lbs.
Steps:
1. Write down the weight in pounds: 150 lbs
2. Use the conversion factor to set up the conversion ratio: 1 kg/2.20462 lbs
3. Multiply the weight in pounds by the conversion ratio to cancel out the lbs unit and get the weight in kg: 150 lbs * 1 kg/2.20462 lbs = 68 kg (rounded to the nearest whole number)

The patient's weight is approximately 68 kg.

Example 2: Converting Medication Dosage from mg to mcg

Medication doses are often written in milligrams (mg), but sometimes, you might need to convert this to micrograms (mcg), especially for very small doses.

Let's say a medication is ordered at 0.125 mg. To convert this to micrograms, we use the conversion factor 1 mg = 1000 mcg.

Steps:
1. Write down the dosage in milligrams: 0.125 mg
2. Use the conversion factor to set up the conversion ratio: 1000 mcg/1 mg
3. Multiply the dosage in mg by the conversion ratio to cancel out the mg unit and get the dosage in mcg: 0.125 mg * 1000 mcg/1 mg = 125 mcg

The medication dosage is 125 mcg.

These examples provide a glimpse of how unit conversions work in healthcare settings. Accuracy in these conversions is vital to ensure safe and effective patient care.

SCIENCE SECTION:

Welcome to the Science Section, a vital component of your ATI TEAS study guide. The fascinating world of science, particularly as it applies to healthcare and nursing, awaits you in this section. As you explore this realm, you'll come to understand how foundational scientific knowledge translates into practical, life-saving applications in a healthcare setting.

Overview

The Science Section is comprised of several key areas:

1. **Human Anatomy and Physiology:** This is the cornerstone of medical science. Understanding the human body's structure (anatomy) and how it functions (physiology) is integral to every aspect of nursing. Here, we'll delve into the various body systems, including the circulatory, respiratory, digestive, nervous, and musculoskeletal systems, among others.
2. **Life and Physical Sciences:** Fundamental principles of biology, chemistry, and physics play a role in our understanding of human health and the practice of medicine. We'll explore cell biology, basic chemical reactions, and physical principles like force and pressure that have direct implications in healthcare.
3. **Scientific Reasoning:** Science is as much a way of thinking as it is a body of knowledge. We'll delve into the scientific method, interpretation of data, and the development of conclusions based on evidence. These skills are not only essential for understanding scientific research but also for making critical decisions in healthcare.

As we navigate through each topic, we'll connect the theoretical aspects with real-world healthcare scenarios to reinforce your understanding and to emphasize the relevance of these scientific concepts in your future nursing practice.

Fasten your seat belts and get ready for a thrilling exploration of the world of science!

The science of nursing is grounded in basic scientific principles. Without a foundational understanding of these principles, a nurse could find it difficult to deliver safe and effective care. Here's why:

1. **Patient Care**: Knowledge of biology and anatomy helps nurses understand how the human body functions in health and disease. This allows them to anticipate a patient's needs, monitor for changes in condition, and understand the rationale behind various treatments.
2. **Medication Administration**: A grasp of chemistry enables nurses to understand how medications interact with the body and with each other. They need to understand things like drug absorption, distribution, metabolism, and excretion, as well as potential drug interactions.
3. **Medical Procedures**: Nurses often need to perform procedures that require a solid understanding of anatomy and physiology, such as placing an IV, administering injections, or performing wound care.
4. **Patient Education**: Nurses play a crucial role in teaching patients about their health conditions and how to manage them. To do this effectively, they need to understand the underlying science.

5. **Evidence-Based Practice**: Modern nursing is grounded in evidence-based practice, which means using the latest scientific research to guide patient care. Understanding the science behind this research is key to applying it effectively.

In short, basic science principles are the foundation of all nursing practice, enabling nurses to provide the best possible care for their patients.

The Science section of the ATI TEAS 7 exam plays a crucial role in evaluating a student's readiness for nursing school, given the integral connection between scientific understanding and competent nursing. In this context, it assesses the breadth and depth of a student's knowledge in key areas that align with the standard pre-nursing school curriculum.

1. **Human Anatomy and Physiology**: A significant portion of the Science section is dedicated to testing a student's understanding of the human body, its organ systems, their functions, and interrelationships. This includes knowledge of basic physical and chemical processes that sustain life, such as respiration, digestion, and circulation.
2. **Biology**: Here, foundational concepts such as cell structure and function, basics of molecular biology, genetics, and evolution are examined. For nursing, a firm grounding in these areas aids in understanding disease processes at a cellular level.
3. **Chemistry**: It is also important for students to grasp basic chemistry concepts, including atomic structure, properties of matter, and chemical reactions. These concepts underpin understanding of various biological processes and the action of different medications and treatments.
4. **Scientific Reasoning**: Lastly, the TEAS Science section tests a student's scientific literacy and reasoning skills, including their ability to interpret scientific data, draw logical conclusions, and apply the scientific method. In the healthcare field, these skills are crucial for evidence-based practice and informed decision-making.

Ultimately, this section evaluates whether students possess the scientific knowledge and understanding that will be built upon in nursing school. A strong performance in this section is a good indicator that a student is prepared to tackle the science-heavy curriculum of nursing school, and subsequently, apply that knowledge in a healthcare setting.

let's delve into the fascinating realm of the human body systems, each playing a critical role in maintaining our overall health and functioning. Here's a brief overview of the primary body systems:

1. **Integumentary System**: This is composed of the skin, hair, and nails. It serves as the body's initial defense against environmental hazards, helps regulate body temperature, and provides sensory information.
2. **Muscular System**: Includes all the muscles of the body. Its primary function is movement, but it also helps maintain posture and produces heat.
3. **Skeletal System**: Composed of bones, cartilage, and ligaments, it provides structural support, facilitates movement, protects vital organs, produces blood cells, and stores minerals.

4. **Nervous System**: Consists of the brain, spinal cord, and nerves. It controls and coordinates body activities, detects and responds to changes in the external and internal environment, and facilitates communication among various body parts.
5. **Endocrine System**: Composed of glands that produce hormones, which are chemical signals sent via the bloodstream to initiate and regulate various body functions like growth, metabolism, and reproduction.
6. **Cardiovascular System**: Includes the heart and blood vessels. It circulates blood, delivering oxygen, nutrients, hormones, and other vital substances to the cells and removing waste products.
7. **Respiratory System**: Comprises the nose, pharynx, larynx, trachea, bronchi, and lungs. It exchanges gases (oxygen and carbon dioxide) between the blood and the air, and helps regulate blood pH.
8. **Digestive System**: Includes the mouth, esophagus, stomach, small and large intestines, and accessory organs like the liver, pancreas, and gallbladder. It breaks down food into nutrients, absorbs those nutrients into the bloodstream, and eliminates indigestible waste.
9. **Urinary System**: Comprises the kidneys, ureters, urinary bladder, and urethra. It filters the blood to remove waste products and excess substances, regulates blood volume and pressure, controls levels of electrolytes and metabolites, and regulates blood pH.
10. **Reproductive System**: Composed of different organs in males (testes, penis, etc.) and females (ovaries, uterus, etc.). It is responsible for producing sex cells and hormones, and in females, it provides for fertilization and development of a new individual.
11. **Lymphatic System**: Consists of lymphatic vessels, lymph nodes, and lymph. It helps maintain fluid balance, absorbs fats from the digestive tract, and helps in the body's defense against disease-causing agents.

Each of these systems contributes to the complex interplay that keeps us alive and well. Understanding these systems and how they interact is vital in nursing, as it aids in assessing, diagnosing, and treating a variety of health conditions.

The human body is like an intricate orchestra, with all of its systems playing together harmoniously to keep us healthy. When one system is out of tune, it can impact the entire symphony of our health. Here's a closer look at how the interconnection of these systems influences health and disease.

1. **Nervous and Endocrine Systems**: The nervous and endocrine systems are heavily interconnected. For instance, stress (a psychological state communicated by the nervous system) can stimulate the adrenal glands (part of the endocrine system) to release hormones like cortisol, which can impact other systems (e.g., suppressing the immune system).
2. **Cardiovascular and Respiratory Systems**: These two systems work in tandem to supply oxygen and remove carbon dioxide from the body. Impairments in one can directly affect the other. For instance, if a person has chronic obstructive pulmonary disease

(COPD), their ability to exchange gases in the lungs is compromised, which can put extra strain on the heart, potentially leading to conditions like right-sided heart failure.
3. **Digestive and Urinary Systems**: These systems collaborate to remove waste from the body. Problems with the digestive system, such as kidney disease, can cause waste products to accumulate in the blood, which can lead to a range of health issues, from high blood pressure to bone disease.
4. **Immune and Integumentary Systems**: The integumentary system serves as the first line of defense against pathogens. If this barrier is compromised (say, by a cut in the skin), the immune system steps up to combat any invaders, preventing infection.
5. **Musculoskeletal and Nervous Systems**: The musculoskeletal system works under the direction of the nervous system to execute movements. Conditions that affect the nervous system, like Parkinson's disease, can severely impact motor function.
6. **Endocrine and Reproductive Systems**: Hormones released by the endocrine system regulate the reproductive system. Imbalances in these hormones can lead to problems like polycystic ovary syndrome (PCOS) or infertility.

In short, the health of one body system can significantly influence the health of others. Understanding these connections allows healthcare professionals to better predict, prevent, and treat various diseases.

Dive into the world of a cell, and you'll find it's like a bustling city, with different parts working together to keep the cell alive and functioning. Here's a brief overview:
1. **Plasma Membrane**: The city limits of our cell, the plasma membrane, is a semi-permeable barrier composed mainly of a double layer of lipids (lipid bilayer), interspersed with proteins. It controls the entry and exit of substances, keeping the cell's internal environment stable.
2. **Cytoplasm**: Within the city limits, you'll find the cytoplasm - a jelly-like substance where all the cellular organelles reside and where most of the cell's metabolic reactions occur.
3. **Nucleus**: The city hall of our cell is the nucleus. It houses the cell's DNA, the genetic blueprint that guides all cell activities. The nucleus is surrounded by a double-membrane nuclear envelope with pores that allow communication with the cytoplasm.
4. **Mitochondria**: These are the power plants of the cell. They generate energy in the form of ATP (adenosine triphosphate) through a process called cellular respiration.
5. **Endoplasmic Reticulum (ER)**: The ER functions as a manufacturing and packaging system. It comes in two varieties: rough ER, studded with ribosomes and involved in protein synthesis, and smooth ER, which is involved in lipid synthesis and detoxification processes.
6. **Golgi Apparatus**: Think of this as the cell's post office. It modifies, sorts, and packages proteins and lipids for transport to their intended destinations.
7. **Lysosomes**: These are the recycling centers. They contain enzymes to digest waste materials and cellular debris.
8. **Ribosomes**: These are the factories where proteins are made, either freely floating in the cytoplasm or attached to the rough ER.

9. **Cytoskeleton**: This gives the cell its shape and structure, like the city's infrastructure. It's composed of microtubules, actin filaments, and intermediate filaments, and it helps with cell movement and intracellular transport.
10. **Centrioles**: These are crucial for cell division, helping to organize the assembly and disassembly of microtubules during the formation of the mitotic spindle.

In this bustling city of life that is a cell, each component has a job to do, ensuring the cell can carry out its functions efficiently. Understanding cellular structure and function is key to a deeper appreciation of how life works on a microscopic level.

Our understanding of genetic material and protein structure has revolutionized modern medicine and continues to have profound implications for healthcare.

Genetics and Personalized Medicine: Knowledge about genes and their associated functions allows us to move toward personalized medicine, an approach where treatment is tailored to the individual. For example, certain genetic variations can make a person more likely to respond positively to a particular medication or more likely to have side effects. A patient's genetic profile can help physicians choose the most effective treatment with the fewest side effects.

Genetic Testing and Disease Prediction: Genetic testing can reveal an individual's predisposition to certain diseases, such as cancer, Alzheimer's, or heart disease. This can lead to early interventions and lifestyle changes that could potentially delay the onset of these conditions or even prevent them entirely.

Gene Therapy: This is a treatment strategy where a patient's genes are manipulated directly to treat or prevent disease. For example, if a patient has a disease caused by a defective gene, a healthy copy of that gene could be introduced to replace the defective one.

Proteomics and Drug Discovery: Proteins are the workhorses of the cell, performing most of the tasks necessary for life. Understanding their structures and functions enables drug developers to create medications that target specific proteins involved in disease processes. This has led to the development of targeted therapies, particularly in the field of cancer treatment.

Understanding Diseases at the Molecular Level: Many diseases, such as cancer and neurodegenerative disorders like Alzheimer's and Parkinson's, involve complex interactions between genes and proteins. By studying these interactions, researchers can gain insights into the mechanisms of these diseases, leading to new treatment strategies.

Vaccines and Biotechnology: Our understanding of genetics and protein structure has allowed us to develop more effective vaccines. For example, the COVID-19 vaccines were developed based on the genetic sequence of the virus, and they instruct our cells to produce a harmless piece of the virus's spike protein to trigger an immune response.

As we continue to delve into the intricate world of genes and proteins, we'll likely continue to see more advancements in medicine that improve patient care and outcomes. This ongoing research is integral to the continuous evolution of healthcare.

let's delve into the fundamentals of atomic structure and its significance in healthcare.

Atoms are the basic building blocks of all matter. They consist of three types of particles: protons, neutrons, and electrons. Protons and neutrons reside in the atom's nucleus (center), while electrons whizz around the nucleus in what's called electron shells.

Protons carry a positive electrical charge, electrons have a negative charge, and neutrons have no charge. The number of protons in an atom determines the atomic number and identifies the element. For instance, hydrogen has one proton, helium has two, and so on.

But why is this relevant in healthcare? Here are a few reasons:

Radiation Therapy: Atomic structure is the foundation of radiation therapy used to treat cancer. Radioactive isotopes, or radionuclides, are used to destroy cancer cells. These are atoms with unstable nuclei that emit radiation, which can damage or destroy cancer cells. Understanding atomic structure allows healthcare professionals to harness this energy safely and effectively.

Diagnostic Imaging: Various imaging techniques, such as MRI, PET, and CT scans, rely on our understanding of atomic structure. For instance, MRI machines work by applying a strong magnetic field that influences the spin of hydrogen atoms in the body. When the magnetic field is turned off, these atoms emit energy signals that are captured and used to create detailed images.

Pharmacology: On a molecular level, the effectiveness of a drug depends on the interactions between the atoms in the drug molecule and the atoms in the body's cells. The atomic structure defines these interactions. In drug design, understanding atomic structure and molecular interactions can help design more effective and safer drugs.

Radiopharmaceuticals: These are medicinal formulations containing radioactive isotopes used in diagnosis and therapy. They work on the principle of radioactive decay, which directly ties back to atomic structure.

These are just a few examples of how a fundamental understanding of atomic structure plays a critical role in healthcare. It helps healthcare providers to understand how treatments work and to make informed decisions regarding patient care.

The properties and changes of matter are integral to numerous physiological processes within the body. To understand this, let's first recall that matter refers to anything that has mass and takes up space. Matter is composed of elements, and these elements combine in various ways to form the multitude of molecules and compounds that make up the human body.

Physical and Chemical Properties of Matter: Matter can be described by its physical properties (such as color, density, and hardness) and chemical properties (how it reacts or changes into other substances). For instance, the fact that water (a key component of the human body) is a liquid at body temperature is a crucial physical property. If water were a gas or a solid at these temperatures, life as we know it would not be possible!

Changes in Matter: Changes in matter can be physical or chemical. Physical changes do not alter the identity of the substance, like when water in the body evaporates into sweat, cooling the skin. Chemical changes, on the other hand, do alter the substance's identity. An example is the breakdown of glucose during cellular respiration, a chemical reaction that provides energy for the body's cells.

Role in Physiological Processes:

1. **Enzymatic Reactions:** Enzymes, which are proteins, catalyze almost all chemical reactions in the body. The unique structure of each enzyme allows it to facilitate specific chemical reactions, turning substrates into products. This is key to processes like digestion and energy production.
2. **Signal Transmission:** Ions, which are atoms with a net electrical charge due to the loss or gain of electrons, play crucial roles in transmitting signals within the body. For example, nerve impulses are transmitted by the movement of sodium and potassium ions across cell membranes.
3. **Gas Exchange:** The physical property of gases to diffuse from areas of high concentration to areas of low concentration is key in the respiratory system. In the lungs, oxygen diffuses from the inhaled air into the blood, while carbon dioxide diffides from the blood into the air to be exhaled.
4. **pH Balance:** The body maintains a stable pH, a measure of acidity or alkalinity, which is essential for all chemical reactions in the body. Various buffer systems prevent drastic changes in pH, protecting the body from harmful shifts in acidity.
5. **Temperature Regulation:** The body maintains a steady internal temperature, an example of thermoregulation, a physical change. This involves both the production of heat, such as through muscle contraction, and the dissipation of heat, through mechanisms like sweating.

Understanding these concepts gives healthcare professionals and medical scientists the knowledge to develop new treatments and interventions, and to understand the effects of diseases and disorders on the body.

Chemical reactions are central to all aspects of human biology and healthcare. From the metabolic processes that give us energy, to the immune response that fights off infections, to the action of medications in our bodies, it's all governed by the principles of chemistry.

Metabolism: At a basic level, the human body is a complex chemical factory. Every cell in our body carries out countless chemical reactions every second. These reactions, known collectively as metabolism, allow us to transform the food we eat into the energy we need to live. For example, the process of cellular respiration is a series of chemical reactions that convert glucose (a simple sugar) and oxygen into water, carbon dioxide, and energy in the form of ATP (adenosine triphosphate).

Drug Action: The development and use of medications are deeply rooted in the principles of chemical reactions. Drugs work by interacting with certain molecules in the body, often by participating in or blocking chemical reactions. For instance, many painkillers work by blocking the chemical reactions that lead to the production of molecules that signal pain to the brain.

Immune Response: Our bodies are constantly fighting off potential threats, such as bacteria and viruses. This is accomplished through a series of complex chemical reactions that allow our immune cells to recognize and destroy these foreign invaders. For example, when a bacterium enters the body, immune cells respond by producing molecules called antibodies that can bind to the bacterium and mark it for destruction.

DNA and Protein Synthesis: The instructions for life are written in the language of DNA, a long molecule made up of a sequence of smaller molecules called nucleotides. When a cell needs to make a protein, it uses a chemical reaction called transcription to create a copy of the relevant DNA sequence in the form of another molecule called RNA. This RNA molecule then undergoes another series of chemical reactions called translation, which converts the RNA sequence into a sequence of amino acids that fold up to form the desired protein.

Regulation of Body Functions: The body maintains its internal environment through a process known as homeostasis, which is governed by a series of chemical reactions. For example, the acidity of our blood is tightly controlled by a chemical buffer system that can neutralize excess acid or base.

Overall, a firm grasp of the principles of chemical reactions not only helps us understand the fundamental processes of life, but also allows healthcare professionals to understand how treatments work, and how different factors can affect patient health.

Scientific measurements and tools form the backbone of healthcare delivery, aiding in everything from basic health assessment to diagnosing complex conditions. The accuracy, precision, and correct use of these tools are paramount to ensuring effective care and patient safety. Let's delve into some examples of how these apply in a healthcare setting.

Thermometers: These tools measure body temperature, a vital sign. Changes in body temperature can signal infection, inflammation, or other health issues. Different types of thermometers, like oral, rectal, ear (tympanic), and forehead (temporal artery) thermometers, may be used based on patient needs and age. Understanding the correct use and interpretation of these tools is essential.

Scales and Measuring Tapes: Weight and height measurements are often taken during patient assessments. They help calculate Body Mass Index (BMI), guide medication dosages, monitor growth in children, and evaluate nutritional status. Nurses also use measuring tapes to measure body parts such as abdominal girth, particularly in cases of swelling or edema.

Sphygmomanometers and Stethoscopes: Used to measure blood pressure, these are crucial tools in detecting and monitoring conditions like hypertension and hypotension. Accurate readings help guide treatment decisions, like the initiation or adjustment of medications. Stethoscopes are also used to listen to heart and lung sounds, which can reveal conditions like murmurs or pneumonia.

Pulse Oximeters: These devices measure oxygen saturation in the blood—a critical measurement for patients with respiratory conditions like COPD, asthma, or COVID-19, or those receiving anesthesia.

Lab Equipment: Various tools are used in laboratory testing, such as microscopes, centrifuges, and pipettes. These allow healthcare professionals to analyze blood, urine, and tissue samples, which can be crucial for diagnosing diseases, identifying infections, or assessing organ function.

Syringes and Infusion Pumps: Syringes are used to deliver precise doses of medication. Infusion pumps regulate the administration of fluids, such as intravenous medications, nutrients, or pain relievers. Precise measurements are crucial to avoid underdosing or overdosing.

Medical Imaging Devices: Tools like X-ray machines, MRI and CT scanners, and ultrasound machines provide internal images of a patient's body. These help diagnose and monitor a vast range of conditions, from fractures to tumors to heart disease.

As you can see, scientific measurements and tools are not just applicable, but absolutely vital in a healthcare setting. Correctly using these tools—and interpreting their readings—enables healthcare professionals to provide the best possible care for their patients.

The scientific method is a systematic way to explore observations and answer questions. It's a structured approach used across the sciences, including healthcare, to ensure consistency and reliability in investigations. Let's walk through the steps of the scientific method and discuss how they're applied in healthcare:

1. **Observation:** This is where it all begins. Healthcare providers make many observations throughout their day. For example, they might notice that a patient's symptoms aren't improving despite the prescribed treatment.
2. **Question:** The observation then leads to a question. Why isn't the treatment working as expected? What might be causing the patient's ongoing symptoms?
3. **Hypothesis:** This is an educated guess about what might be happening, based on previous knowledge and the specific observation. In our example, the healthcare provider might hypothesize that the patient has an undiagnosed condition that's interfering with treatment.
4. **Experiment:** To test the hypothesis, an experiment or investigation is conducted. This might involve additional diagnostic tests, a review of the patient's medical history, or a trial of a different treatment approach.
5. **Data Collection and Analysis:** The healthcare provider collects and analyzes data from the experiment. This could involve tracking the patient's symptoms, measuring response to treatment, or interpreting results from diagnostic tests.
6. **Conclusion:** Based on the data, the healthcare provider draws a conclusion. The conclusion might support the initial hypothesis, or it might contradict it, leading to a new hypothesis and more experiments.
7. **Communication:** Findings are communicated to other members of the healthcare team, the patient, and potentially, the wider medical community. This could involve documenting the patient's response in their medical record, discussing the case with colleagues, or even publishing the findings in a medical journal if the case adds to understanding of a particular condition or treatment approach.

In healthcare, the scientific method is used daily in diagnosis and treatment decisions. It guides research to develop new treatments, improve patient care, and increase understanding of health and disease. Moreover, it's a key tool for healthcare providers in troubleshooting when a patient's health issue isn't responding to standard approaches. By using this structured approach, healthcare professionals can ensure that their decisions are based on evidence and careful analysis, ultimately leading to better patient outcomes.

ENGLISH AND LANGUAGE USAGE SECTION:

Welcome to the English and Language Usage Section chapter of our ATI TEAS 7 prep guide. In this comprehensive section, we aim to provide a thorough overview of all the essential concepts, tools, and skills that you will need to perform well in this portion of the ATI TEAS 7 exam.

The English and Language Usage section of the exam evaluates your ability to effectively use the English language, which is crucial for success in any nursing program. This part of the TEAS test evaluates your knowledge and skills in several key areas such as vocabulary, grammar, punctuation, sentence structure, contextual words, and spelling. It also assesses your ability to comprehend and analyze a variety of written materials.

This chapter is structured in a way that allows you to delve deep into each aspect of the English language, beginning with an understanding of vocabulary, and proceeding into the nuances of grammar, sentence structure, and language conventions. We also touch upon the aspects of understanding and interpreting a variety of texts, a skill fundamental to following complex medical instructions, interpreting patient information, and understanding healthcare literature.

Our aim is not only to prepare you for the test but also to ensure that you're equipped with the communication skills necessary for a successful nursing career. Each concept is explained in a clear, concise manner with practical examples, and is accompanied by useful tips and strategies to help you answer questions accurately and quickly.

Let's embark on this linguistic journey together, enhancing your language skills and boosting your confidence for the English and Language Usage section of the ATI TEAS 7 exam.

The English and Language Usage section of the ATI TEAS 7 exam assesses a student's knowledge and skills in the areas of grammar, sentence structure, punctuation, and spelling. This section is an integral part of the examination as it evaluates the readiness of the candidate to comprehend and effectively communicate in English, a fundamental requirement for success in any nursing program.

This section is structured into several sub-areas:

1. **Conventions of Standard English**: This sub-section focuses on grammar, sentence structure, and punctuation. It assesses the ability of the candidate to apply the conventions of standard English, which is crucial for clear and effective communication in a healthcare setting.
2. **Knowledge of Language**: This sub-area tests the understanding of language and the use of various techniques to convey and comprehend messages accurately. It often includes questions about context and implication, tonal shifts, and more complex language structures.

3. **Vocabulary Acquisition**: This sub-section gauges the ability to use various strategies to determine the meaning of words and phrases. It tests knowledge of common medical terminologies and the capacity to understand and interpret complex vocabulary in context.
4. **Spelling**: This is the component that tests the ability of the candidate to spell words correctly. Spelling can impact clarity and credibility in written communication, so this skill is important.

The English and Language Usage section, like the other sections of the ATI TEAS 7 exam, requires a comprehensive understanding and proficient use of English. This is essential as nurses must be able to effectively communicate with their patients, doctors, and other healthcare professionals, making this section vital for their future careers.

Vocabulary is incredibly important in nursing for a variety of reasons. At its core, it forms the basis for communication between healthcare professionals and between caregivers and patients. Let's dive into some details:
1. **Clear Communication**: A solid grasp of vocabulary allows for precise and effective communication. In healthcare, miscommunication or misunderstanding can have serious consequences, so clear communication is critical.
2. **Professionalism**: Knowledge of professional vocabulary demonstrates competence and helps to build trust with colleagues, patients, and their families.
3. **Efficiency**: The use of specific medical terms can convey a lot of information quickly and succinctly. It makes communication more efficient, which is especially important in time-sensitive situations.
4. **Patient Care**: Understanding medical terms helps in interpreting patients' symptoms, medical histories, and treatment plans accurately.

Now, let's look at some examples of commonly used terms in nursing:
- **Ambulatory**: Refers to a patient who is able to walk.
- **Biopsy**: A procedure that involves taking a small piece of body tissue to examine it more closely.
- **Catheter**: A tube used to drain fluids from or administer fluids to the body.
- **Dyspnea**: Difficulty or discomfort when breathing.
- **Edema**: Swelling caused by an excess of fluid in the tissues.
- **Hemorrhage**: Excessive or uncontrolled bleeding.
- **Intravenous (IV)**: Into a vein. Often used to refer to the method of administering medication or fluids directly into a vein.
- **Prognosis**: The likely course or outcome of a disease.
- **Sepsis**: A serious and potentially life-threatening response to infection, leading to organ dysfunction.
- **Vital signs**: Clinical measurements that indicate the body's basic functions, including temperature, pulse, breathing rate, and blood pressure.

These are just a few examples, but they demonstrate the variety and specificity of medical vocabulary. Remember, a comprehensive understanding of these terms is essential for delivering high-quality care in a nursing career.

Understanding grammar rules and conventions is essential for clear, effective communication, particularly in a healthcare setting. Misunderstandings can have serious implications, so the precision and clarity that comes with good grammar is vital. Let's consider a few reasons why:

1. **Clarity**: Proper grammar helps to ensure that the intended message is received without confusion or misinterpretation. This can be particularly crucial in healthcare, where complex and nuanced information is often being conveyed.
2. **Professionalism**: Adherence to grammatical rules is seen as a marker of professionalism. It aids in maintaining a level of formality and respect in communication.
3. **Documentation**: Healthcare settings often involve a significant amount of documentation, such as patient records, treatment plans, and diagnostic reports. Good grammar helps to ensure that these documents are clear and understandable to all who read them, which can include a diverse range of healthcare professionals.
4. **Patient Care**: Good grammar can also improve patient care by facilitating clear communication between the healthcare provider and the patient. This can help to ensure that the patient fully understands their health situation and the proposed treatments.
5. **Interprofessional Communication**: In healthcare, you often collaborate with a variety of professionals, including doctors, pharmacists, physiotherapists, social workers, and more. Precise grammar allows for more effective interdisciplinary communication, which can lead to improved patient outcomes.

Therefore, understanding grammar rules and conventions is not just about "correctness" for its own sake, but is a tool to enhance communication, promote professionalism, and ultimately, to support the delivery of effective healthcare.

A strong foundation in sentence structure is crucial for clear and effective communication. Understanding how sentences are constructed is akin to knowing the blueprint of a building – it allows you to construct your own sentences accurately and comprehend others' messages more effectively.

Sentence structure, at its most basic level, is built around two core parts: the subject and the predicate. The subject refers to what or whom the sentence is about, while the predicate expresses what is being said about the subject. It usually contains a verb, and it may also include objects or complements.

For example, in the sentence "The nurse administers the medication," "The nurse" is the subject, and "administers the medication" is the predicate. The action (verb) is "administers," and the object of the action is "the medication."

But that's not all. Sentences can be made more complex with the addition of phrases and clauses. A phrase is a group of words that act as a single unit but lack either a subject or a verb (for example, "with a smile"). A clause, on the other hand, is a group of words containing both a subject and a verb, and it can be either independent (able to stand alone as a sentence) or dependent (requiring an independent clause to form a complete sentence).

Mastering sentence structure allows healthcare professionals to communicate more effectively. Clarity of communication is particularly important in healthcare settings, where miscommunications can lead to misunderstandings or errors in patient care. For instance, when writing patient reports, nurses need to be precise and concise, leaving no room for ambiguity. Similarly, in speaking with patients, clear sentence structure helps ensure that instructions and information are understood correctly. Thus, understanding sentence structure is vital not just for the TEAS exam, but for the entirety of your future healthcare career.

Punctuation, in essence, is a system of symbols that we use to structure and organize our writing. It plays a central role in written communication by clarifying the meaning of sentences, managing the pace of the text, and helping to convey the writer's tone or mood.
Let's delve into some of the key punctuation marks and their roles:

1. Periods (.) are used to mark the end of a sentence. They signal a full stop and indicate that a complete thought or statement has been made.
2. Commas (,) have several uses. They can separate items in a list, set off nonessential information, signal a pause within a sentence, and separate independent clauses when used with a coordinating conjunction (for, and, nor, but, or, yet, so).
3. Semicolons (;) are used to connect closely related independent clauses in a single sentence, providing a break that's longer than a comma but shorter than a period.
4. Colons (:) are used to introduce a list, a quote, or an explanation that follows a complete sentence.
5. Question marks (?) are used at the end of a sentence to indicate a direct question.
6. Exclamation marks (!) are used to indicate strong emotion or emphasis.
7. Quotation marks (" ") are used to enclose direct quotations or the titles of short works like articles or poems.
8. Apostrophes (') show possession (e.g., the patient's chart) and are used in contractions to replace missing letters (e.g., it's for it is).
9. Parentheses ( ) and dashes (--) can be used to include additional, often nonessential, information within a sentence.

In the healthcare field, correct punctuation is crucial because it ensures clear and precise communication. For example, the placement of a comma can change the meaning of a sentence, which could have significant consequences in healthcare communication. Consider the difference between "Let's eat, grandma" and "Let's eat grandma." Without proper punctuation, the message can be drastically misinterpreted. Hence, a firm grasp of punctuation rules will not only help you succeed in the TEAS exam but also enhance your professional communication skills.

Understanding and using contextual words are essential skills in English language usage. This involves being able to determine the meaning of words and phrases based on how they are used within a specific context. Here are some strategies to do so:

1. **Identify Clues within the Sentence:** Pay attention to the words around the unfamiliar word. For example, words like 'and', 'or', 'but', and 'while' can provide clues about whether the unknown word has a similar meaning, an additional meaning, an opposing meaning, or a contrasting meaning to the other words in the sentence.
2. **Look for Synonyms and Antonyms:** Sometimes, the context may directly provide a synonym (a word with a similar meaning) or antonym (a word with the opposite meaning) to the unfamiliar word.
3. **Understand the Tone and Setting:** The overall tone and setting of the text can also provide clues about the meaning of the word. For instance, a word in a medical report may have a different connotation than when used in a casual conversation.
4. **Use Word Parts:** Breaking the word down into its root, prefixes, and suffixes can often hint at its meaning. For example, in healthcare, the prefix 'cardio-' refers to the heart, so even if you don't know what 'cardiology' means, you could guess it has something to do with the heart.
5. **Apply Your Knowledge:** Use your background knowledge about the topic at hand. If you're reading a text about nursing, your understanding of nursing practices might help you guess the meaning of unfamiliar terms.
6. **Guess and Check:** Make an educated guess about the meaning of the word based on the context, then look up the word to check if your guess was correct. This active engagement can help reinforce learning.

Remember, the TEAS exam and healthcare settings will both require understanding of specialized vocabulary. So, using context to understand new words is a critical skill to develop. It allows for better comprehension of study materials, more accurate interpretation of exam questions and, in the long run, more effective communication in the healthcare field.

Spelling correctly is crucial for clear and professional communication, especially in the healthcare industry where a single spelling mistake could lead to misinterpretation of vital information. Here are some common spelling rules and tips for remembering difficult spellings:

1. **I before E, except after C:** This classic spelling rule is a handy reminder that 'i' usually comes before 'e' in a word, like 'piece', but after a 'c', it's the other way around, like in 'receive'. Keep in mind, though, this rule has exceptions, such as 'weird' or 'seize'.
2. **Silent E:** If a word ends with a silent 'e', drop the 'e' before adding a suffix that begins with a vowel, such as '-ing' or '-able'. For example, 'write' becomes 'writing' and 'manage' becomes 'manageable'. But keep the 'e' when the suffix starts with a consonant, like 'management'.
3. **Double Consonants:** In general, if a word ends in a single vowel and a consonant, and the stress is on the last syllable, you double the final consonant before adding a suffix. So, 'stop' becomes 'stopping', and 'begin' turns into 'beginning'. But 'visit' stays 'visiting', because the stress is not on the last syllable.

4. **Plural Forms:** Most words simply add an 's' to make them plural, but words that end in 'y' preceded by a consonant change the 'y' to 'i' and add 'es'. So, 'baby' becomes 'babies'. And remember, words ending in 'f' or 'fe' often change to 'ves', like 'wolf' to 'wolves'.
5. **Mnemonics:** Use mnemonic devices to remember difficult spellings. For example, to remember that 'separate' has 'a rat' in the middle, you might picture a rat separating two pieces of cheese.
6. **Word Breakdown:** Break the word into smaller parts or syllables and learn each part individually. It's easier to remember 'in-tel-li-gent' rather than 'intelligent' as a whole.
7. **Constant Practice:** Regularly reading and writing helps reinforce correct spelling. Flashcards, spelling quizzes, and spelling games can also be effective tools.

Spelling can be tricky with all its exceptions and irregularities, but these rules and strategies can help build a strong foundation. In the context of the TEAS exam and nursing practice, accurate spelling is crucial for effective communication and ensuring patient safety.

In the realm of nursing, the ability to comprehend and analyze a wide variety of written materials is absolutely integral to the delivery of effective and safe patient care.

Firstly, every patient comes with their unique medical history, test results, doctor's notes, and care plans - all documented in written form. Nurses need to accurately interpret these records to understand the patient's health status and the prescribed treatment regimen.

Secondly, nursing is a field that's continually evolving with new research and practices. Nurses regularly review scientific literature, articles, and research studies to stay abreast of the latest advancements and improve their practice. Their ability to comprehend these often complex texts can lead to better patient outcomes.

Additionally, written communication is pivotal in nursing. Nurses must record patient symptoms, reactions to medications, and progress in medical charts. Clear, precise, and accurate recording ensures seamless continuity of care among the healthcare team.

Moreover, nurses often have to understand and explain complex medical information to patients and their families in a comprehensible manner. By accurately interpreting written materials, they can effectively translate that information, enhancing patient understanding, cooperation, and satisfaction.

Finally, comprehension and analysis skills are essential for legal and ethical reasons. Nurses must understand hospital policies, legal documents, and ethical guidelines to ensure they uphold the standards of their profession and protect their patients' rights.

In summary, the ability to comprehend and analyze written materials is not just a tool for passing the TEAS; it's a vital skill for successful and impactful nursing practice.

Here are some examples of the types of questions you might encounter in the English and Language Usage section of the ATI TEAS 7 exam:
1. **Spelling:** You might be asked to identify the correct spelling of a word or to choose the misspelled word in a given sentence. For example, "Which of the following words is spelled incorrectly: a) necessary, b) independant, c) recommend, d) occurrence?"
2. **Grammar:** You may encounter questions that require you to select the grammatically correct sentence or to identify the sentence with a grammatical error. An example might be, "Which of the following sentences uses correct subject-verb agreement: a) The team of doctors are arriving, b) The team of doctors is arriving?"
3. **Punctuation:** You could be asked to identify the sentence with the correct punctuation. For instance, "Select the sentence that uses commas correctly: a) I need to buy bread, milk and, eggs, b) I need to buy bread, milk, and eggs."
4. **Sentence Structure:** Questions may require you to recognize complete sentences, sentence fragments, or run-on sentences. A question could look like this: "Which of the following is a complete sentence: a) Running in the park, b) I enjoy running in the park?"
5. **Vocabulary and Contextual Words:** You might be asked to determine the meaning of a word based on the context or to choose a word that best fits in a sentence. An example might be, "In the context of this sentence, what does the word 'ample' most closely mean: 'The hospital provided ample resources for patient care.'"
6. **Paragraph and Passage Comprehension:** Some questions will present a short passage, followed by questions related to its main idea, supporting details, or inferences that can be drawn from it. For example, "What is the main idea of the following passage...?"

Remember, each question tests your knowledge of English language conventions and your ability to effectively apply these rules in different contexts. It's important to read each question carefully and consider each answer choice before making your selection.

Here are some effective strategies to improve both speed and accuracy in the English and Language Usage section of the ATI TEAS 7 exam:
1. **Understand the basics:** Build a solid foundation of grammar, punctuation, and spelling rules. Having a good grasp of these fundamental rules can dramatically increase your speed, as you won't waste time trying to remember them during the test.
2. **Practice active reading:** When reading comprehension questions appear, don't just passively read the text. Highlight key points, take brief notes, and try to summarize what you're reading. Active engagement can enhance your understanding and help you answer questions more accurately.
3. **Master vocabulary:** Regularly expand your vocabulary and understand the usage of words in different contexts. This can not only help with direct vocabulary questions, but also aid in reading comprehension and sentence completion tasks.
4. **Answer easier questions first:** If you come across a question that seems too difficult, skip it and move on to the next. This helps to prevent getting stuck and wasting valuable

time on a single question. You can always come back to the more challenging questions once you've answered the ones you're confident about.
5. **Use process of elimination:** If you're unsure about an answer, start by eliminating the options you know are incorrect. This narrows down the possible correct answers and increases your chances of choosing the right one.
6. **Practice, Practice, Practice:** The more you practice, the more familiar you'll become with the types of questions on the test. Use practice tests to get a feel for the pacing of the exam and to build your confidence.
7. **Mind your time:** Keep an eye on the clock and try to pace yourself. If you're spending too long on one question, it's better to make an educated guess and move on, rather than risk not completing the section.

Remember, preparation is key. By using these strategies during your study and on test day, you can improve both your speed and accuracy in the English and Language Usage section.

Clear and effective communication plays a crucial role in healthcare settings, influencing everything from patient care to the coordination between healthcare professionals. Here's why:
1. **Patient Understanding:** Patients must comprehend their health status, treatment options, and necessary lifestyle changes. If a healthcare provider communicates effectively, it can enhance a patient's understanding and compliance with medical advice.
2. **Patient Safety:** Miscommunication can lead to errors in diagnosis, treatment, and medication administration. By communicating effectively, healthcare providers can minimize errors, ensure patient safety, and enhance the quality of care.
3. **Empathy and Trust:** Good communication helps build trust and empathy. When a patient feels heard and understood, it can improve their satisfaction and engagement in their care. They're also more likely to follow through with treatments and report any issues promptly.
4. **Interprofessional Collaboration:** Healthcare is a collaborative field, involving numerous professionals from various specialties. Clear communication within this team is critical to ensure seamless and comprehensive care for patients. It can help in coordinating responsibilities, discussing patient progress, and making collective decisions.
5. **Informed Consent:** In healthcare, informed consent is a vital ethical and legal requirement. Providers must clearly explain procedures, risks, benefits, and alternatives to patients. Effective communication ensures the patient fully understands this information, which enables them to make informed decisions about their care.
6. **Health Literacy:** Not all patients have the same level of health literacy. Clear, simple, and jargon-free communication can help bridge this gap and ensure that patients understand their health conditions and the prescribed care plan.
7. **Cultural Competence:** Healthcare providers often serve diverse populations. Understanding and respecting cultural differences, including communication norms, is key to providing culturally competent care.

Thus, clear and effective communication is not merely an additional skill but a necessity in healthcare. It's pivotal in ensuring patient safety, satisfaction, and the overall quality of care. The ability to communicate effectively is an essential competency that healthcare professionals, including nurses, must continually develop.

Understanding language usage is central to providing quality patient care in multiple ways:
1. **Effective Communication:** Proficiency in language usage allows healthcare providers to clearly articulate diagnoses, treatment plans, and health education. This leads to enhanced patient understanding, compliance, and ultimately better health outcomes.
2. **Active Listening:** Understanding language usage isn't only about speaking; it's also about effective listening. Recognizing cues in a patient's language can help identify their concerns, fears, or symptoms that they may not explicitly mention.
3. **Empathy and Trust:** A sensitive use of language can demonstrate empathy, helping to build trust and rapport with patients. This trust can encourage patients to be more open about their symptoms and health history, leading to more accurate diagnoses and personalized care plans.
4. **Cultural Competence:** Healthcare providers serve diverse populations with varying languages and dialects. Understanding the nuances of language usage can improve cultural competence and ensure that healthcare services are respectful of and responsive to diverse cultural health beliefs and practices.
5. **Interprofessional Communication:** Clear language usage is also crucial in communicating with other healthcare professionals. It allows for the efficient exchange of patient information, coordination of care, and team collaboration.
6. **Documentation:** Language proficiency is crucial for precise, clear, and succinct documentation in patient records, ensuring continuity of care and reducing errors.
7. **Health Education:** Healthcare providers often need to educate patients about their health conditions and preventive measures. Understanding language usage can assist in conveying complex medical information in a way that's easy for patients to understand, enabling them to take active roles in their health.

In sum, a deep understanding of language usage facilitates better communication, promotes patient-centered care, and improves health outcomes. It's an essential skill for anyone in the healthcare field, especially nurses, who often serve as the primary point of contact for patients.

Here are a few examples of exercises or practice questions that can help you prepare for the English and Language Usage section of the ATI TEAS 7 exam:
1. **Grammar Practice:**
    - Identify the grammatical errors in the following sentence: "The patients is happy because their symptoms has improved."
    - Select the correct verb form for the sentence: "Each of the nurses _____ (has/have) a unique approach to patient care."
2. **Punctuation Practice:**

- Rewrite the following sentence with the correct punctuation: "The doctor said the patient's progress is remarkable she is recovering faster than expected."
- Place commas in the correct places in this sentence: "When the patient arrives tomorrow at 3 pm I will be ready to perform the examination."

3. **Spelling Practice:**
   - Correct the spelling errors in the sentence: "The phlebotomist collected a vial of blud for testing."
   - Identify the misspelled word: "The pediatrician provided comprehensive care to the patiant."

4. **Contextual Words:**
   - Choose the correct word to complete the sentence: "The nurse needed to remain (stationary/stationery) while monitoring the patient's vital signs."
   - Fill in the blank: "The surgeon was _____ (averse/advert) to performing the operation due to the patient's high risk factors."

5. **Reading Comprehension:**
   - Given a paragraph from a nursing textbook or a patient case history, answer questions like: "What is the main idea of this passage?" or "What can be inferred from the patient's symptoms?"

These types of exercises can help you build proficiency in the English and Language Usage section. However, remember that consistent practice and a thorough understanding of the concepts are the keys to success on the exam.

EXAM PREP SECTION:

Welcome to the practice exam section! This part of the book is designed to provide you with a practical and comprehensive approach to preparing for the ATI TEAS 7 exam. We understand the importance of practice in familiarizing yourself with the structure of the exam and the types of questions you're likely to encounter. That's why we've included a diverse range of practice questions in this section to help you fine-tune your skills and build your confidence.

Now, you may notice something different in our practice exam section - the answer to each question is provided immediately after the question. We've chosen this unique layout for several reasons.

Firstly, we want to provide immediate feedback on your responses. This approach allows you to actively learn and adjust your understanding in real-time, fostering deeper comprehension and more robust learning. The mind is most receptive to learning directly after a question has been attempted, making this the perfect time to provide the answer.

Secondly, having the answer and an explanation right after the question eliminates the need to flip back and forth to an answer key at the back of the book. This saves time and makes for a smoother, more focused study experience. You can stay immersed in the subject matter without unnecessary interruptions.

Lastly, our explanations aren't just there to justify the correct answer. They also provide additional insights and help clarify common misconceptions, acting as miniature lessons in themselves. By understanding the rationale behind each answer, you're not just memorizing the right choice—you're comprehending why it's the right choice.

As you work through this section, remember that practice is a process. Your performance on these questions today is not a final verdict, but a step on your journey towards mastering the material. Embrace each question as an opportunity to learn and improve. Let's begin!

Test-taking strategies and study tips are essential for successfully navigating the ATI TEAS 7 exam. Here are some strategies to keep in mind:
1. **Develop a Study Plan:** Plan your study schedule well in advance of your test date. Identify the times of the day when you study best and make that your regular study time.
2. **Focus on Understanding, not Memorizing:** Understanding concepts deeply will be more beneficial than just memorizing facts. This will also help you answer application-based questions that test your understanding of concepts.
3. **Practice Regularly:** Regular practice with test questions can improve your familiarity with the format of the exam and reduce test anxiety. Using official ATI TEAS practice materials can be especially helpful.
4. **Use the Process of Elimination:** On multiple choice questions, use the process of elimination to narrow down your options. This strategy can increase your chances of choosing the correct answer.

5. **Manage Your Time:** The ATI TEAS exam is timed, so it's important to keep a steady pace. Don't spend too much time on any one question. If you're stuck, make an educated guess and move on.
6. **Read Questions Carefully:** Make sure to read each question and all the answer choices thoroughly before selecting your answer. Misunderstanding the question is a common mistake.
7. **Use All Available Resources:** While studying, use the resources available to you, such as textbooks, online resources, study guides, flashcards, and group study sessions. Diversifying your study materials can help reinforce learning.
8. **Stay Healthy:** Regular exercise, a balanced diet, and plenty of sleep are all important for optimal brain function. Don't neglect your physical health while studying.
9. **Stay Positive and Reduce Stress:** Maintaining a positive attitude and managing stress are also important. Remember to take breaks during study sessions and do activities that help you relax and recharge.
10. **Review, Review, Review:** Regularly revisit material you've studied in the past. The more often you review, the better you'll retain the information.

Remember, the key to doing well on any exam is preparation. The more effort you put into preparing for the ATI TEAS 7 exam, the more confident you'll be on test day.

Test anxiety is a common issue, but there are strategies to manage it effectively, especially in the context of the ATI TEAS exam:
1. **Understand the Format**: Familiarize yourself with the format of the ATI TEAS exam. Knowing what to expect can help alleviate fear of the unknown. Review the structure, types of questions, and time limits for each section.
2. **Plan and Prepare**: Create a consistent study schedule leading up to the exam. Cramming the night before can increase anxiety. Break down the material into manageable chunks and review regularly to solidify your understanding.
3. **Take Practice Exams**: This can help you get used to the test format and timing. Additionally, analyzing your performance on practice tests can help you identify areas where you need to focus your study efforts.
4. **Stay Healthy**: Regular exercise, a balanced diet, and adequate sleep can reduce physical symptoms of anxiety. Avoid caffeine and sugar before the exam, as these can increase feelings of nervousness.
5. **Practice Relaxation Techniques**: Techniques such as deep breathing, progressive muscle relaxation, and visualization can help you stay calm and focused. Find what works best for you and practice it regularly, both during study sessions and in the exam.
6. **Develop a Positive Mindset**: Negative self-talk can increase anxiety. Instead, try to cultivate a positive mindset. Remind yourself of your preparation and ability to tackle the test.
7. **Arrive Early**: Plan to arrive at the test center early. This can prevent last-minute rushing, which can exacerbate anxiety.
8. **Read Carefully**: Take the time to carefully read each question and each answer choice before making a decision. Rushing through the test can lead to mistakes and increase anxiety.
9. **Take Short Breaks**: During the exam, if you find your anxiety rising, close your eyes, take a few deep breaths, and then return to the test. This brief break can help you regain your composure.
10. **Seek Support**: If test anxiety is seriously impacting your ability to prepare for or take the ATI TEAS, consider seeking support from a counselor or mental health professional. They can provide strategies and resources to manage anxiety effectively.

Remember, it's normal to feel some level of anxiety before a test—it can even be motivating. But if it becomes overwhelming, these strategies can help manage your stress and perform your best on the ATI TEAS exam.

Using the process of elimination can be a vital strategy while taking the ATI TEAS exam. This tactic can help you arrive at the correct answer by ruling out the incorrect ones. Here's how to effectively use this strategy:

1. **Read the Entire Question First**: Before glancing at the answer choices, make sure you fully understand what the question is asking. Sometimes, the question itself may contain hints that can help you eliminate certain options.
2. **Review Each Answer Choice**: Read each option carefully. Do not rush to select the first answer that seems right. Instead, consider all options before making your decision.
3. **Cross Out Clearly Incorrect Answers**: In some cases, it will be apparent that certain answers are incorrect. They may contradict the information given in the question, be factually wrong, or be irrelevant to the question asked. If you're sure an answer choice is incorrect, mentally cross it out.
4. **Look for Extremes**: If an answer choice includes absolute terms like 'always,' 'never,' 'all,' or 'none,' it may be incorrect. Few things in life are absolute, and this is especially true in nursing and healthcare. However, use this rule with caution, as it doesn't always hold true.
5. **Trust Your Gut**: If two options seem possible but one feels more likely to you based on your studies and understanding of the subject, consider choosing that one.
6. **Guess Wisely**: If you've eliminated one or two choices, and you're still unsure of the answer, it's better to make an educated guess rather than leave the question blank. With fewer options to choose from, your chances of selecting the correct answer increases.

Remember, the process of elimination is just one of the strategies you can use when taking the ATI TEAS exam. Combining it with other tactics such as time management, understanding the format of the test, and preparing thoroughly can help increase your chances of success.

In the context of the ATI TEAS exam, making educated guesses is an essential skill that can help you navigate tricky questions or those that leave you stumped. It's important to remember that there's no penalty for guessing on this exam, meaning you won't lose points for incorrect answers. Therefore, it's always better to guess than to leave a question blank. Here's how to make educated guesses more effectively:

1. **Eliminate Incorrect Choices**: Use the process of elimination to cross out any answer choices that are clearly incorrect. This approach narrows down your options and increases the likelihood that your guess will be correct.
2. **Identify Patterns or Connections**: Look for relationships between the question and the answer choices. This might involve recalling related concepts or terms that you've studied.
3. **Beware of Absolute Language**: Answer choices that use words like "always," "never," "all," or "none" can often be incorrect because they leave no room for exceptions. However, this isn't a hard and fast rule, so use your discretion.
4. **Trust Your Instincts**: Your first instinct is often correct, especially if you've been diligent in your studies. If you're torn between two choices and time is running out, it's typically best to go with your gut.
5. **Look for the Longest Answer**: While this isn't a foolproof method, sometimes the longest answer is correct because test makers need to ensure the correct answer is indisputably right. Therefore, they might include more qualifiers or detail.

6. **Consider Common Themes**: If you notice that several questions in a row have had the same answer, be wary. It's unlikely that every answer will be "B", for example.

Remember, guessing should not be your main strategy, but it can help when you encounter questions that you're unsure about. Thorough preparation and understanding of the material will always be your best bet for success on the ATI TEAS exam.

1. In a passage about the history of transportation, the author writes, "In the 1800s, the advent of the steam engine revolutionized travel. Distances that once took weeks to traverse could now be covered in a matter of days." Based on the passage, the word "advent" most likely means:
a) Decline
b) Journey
c) Introduction
d) Problem

Answer: c) Introduction
Explanation: In this context, "advent" refers to the appearance or arrival of something significant or noteworthy. The passage tells us that travel changed dramatically with the "advent" of the steam engine, suggesting that this was a new development in the 1800s.

2. The main idea of a passage can often be found:
a) Only in the first sentence of the passage.
b) Dispersed throughout the entire text.
c) Within the conclusion paragraph.
d) Any of the above.

Answer: d) Any of the above
Explanation: The main idea of a passage can be located in different places depending on the writing style of the author. Sometimes it's in the first sentence, serving as a thesis statement. Other times, it might be concluded at the end, or be inferred from information spread throughout the text.

3. When reading a passage about an unfamiliar topic, what strategy can be most helpful for comprehension?
a) Skipping the difficult parts
b) Looking for context clues to understand new vocabulary
c) Focusing only on the familiar information
d) Reading the passage as quickly as possible

Answer: b) Looking for context clues to understand new vocabulary
Explanation: When you encounter unfamiliar words or concepts, context clues—information from the words or sentences around it—can help you decipher their meaning. This strategy enhances your comprehension of the text as a whole.

4. In a healthcare setting, which type of document would most likely include instructions for patient care?
a) Administrative record
b) Employee handbook
c) Health insurance claim
d) Medical protocol

Answer: d) Medical protocol
Explanation: Medical protocols typically contain guidelines for patient care. They provide healthcare professionals with the steps they should follow in various medical situations.

5. Which of the following is NOT a purpose of a persuasive text?
a) To entertain
b) To convince
c) To argue
d) To influence

Answer: a) To entertain
Explanation: Persuasive texts are written with the goal of convincing the reader to accept a particular viewpoint or take a certain action. While they might occasionally entertain, their main objective is not entertainment but rather to argue, convince, or influence.

6. Passage 1: "Solar energy has been used by humans for thousands of years. Using sunlight for heating water and homes was a common practice in ancient Greece and Rome. Today, it is becoming a significant source of energy for many people around the world. The energy from the sun is sustainable, abundant, and free, making it an attractive alternative to fossil fuels."

What is the main idea of this passage?
a. Ancient Greece and Rome used solar energy.
b. Solar energy is a significant source of energy for many people around the world.
c. Solar energy is sustainable, abundant, and free.
d. The sun's energy is an attractive alternative to fossil fuels.

Answer: b. Solar energy is a significant source of energy for many people around the world.
Explanation: While all the options are points made in the passage, the main idea that ties everything together is that solar energy is a significant source of energy for many people. The passage provides a historical background and benefits, supporting the main idea.

7. Passage 2: "Running is a popular form of exercise that comes with numerous health benefits. It can increase cardiovascular fitness, build strong bones, and help maintain a healthy weight. Despite the physical demand, the simplicity of running makes it a widely accessible activity for people of all ages."

What is the main idea of the passage?
a. Running can increase cardiovascular fitness.
b. Running builds strong bones.
c. Running can help maintain a healthy weight.
d. Running is a simple and accessible form of exercise with various health benefits.

Answer: d. Running is a simple and accessible form of exercise with various health benefits.
Explanation: The other options are supporting details that contribute to the main idea that running is a simple and accessible form of exercise with various health benefits.

8. Passage 3: "Trees play a critical role in maintaining Earth's ecosystem. They not only produce oxygen and provide habitats for animals but also offer shade, prevent soil erosion, and combat climate change by absorbing carbon dioxide."

What is the main idea of this passage?
a. Trees produce oxygen.
b. Trees offer shade and prevent soil erosion.
c. Trees combat climate change by absorbing carbon dioxide.
d. Trees play a critical role in maintaining Earth's ecosystem.

Answer: d. Trees play a critical role in maintaining Earth's ecosystem.
Explanation: While the passage discusses several benefits of trees, the main idea is that they play a critical role in maintaining Earth's ecosystem.

9. Passage 4: "A healthy diet is essential for good health and nutrition. It protects against many chronic noncommunicable diseases, like heart disease, diabetes, and cancer. Eating a variety of foods and consuming less salt, sugars, and saturated and industrially-produced trans-fats, are essential for a healthy diet."

What is the main idea of the passage?
a. A healthy diet protects against many chronic noncommunicable diseases.
b. Eating a variety of foods is essential for a healthy diet.
c. Consuming less salt, sugars, and saturated and industrially-produced trans-fats, are essential for a healthy diet.
d. A healthy diet is essential for good health and nutrition.

Answer: d. A healthy diet is essential for good health and nutrition.
Explanation: The main idea of the passage is that a healthy diet is essential for good health and nutrition. The other options are supporting details that explain why a healthy diet is important.

10. Passage 5: "Mental health is as crucial as physical health. It impacts our thoughts, behaviors, and emotions. Good mental health allows people to realize their full potential, cope with the stresses of life, work productively, and contribute to their communities."

What is the main idea of the passage?
a. Mental health impacts our thoughts, behaviors, and emotions.
b. Good mental health allows people to realize their full potential.
c. People with good mental health can work productively.
d. Mental health is as crucial as physical health.

Answer: d. Mental health is as crucial as physical health.
Explanation: While the passage discusses several aspects of mental health, the main idea is that mental health is as crucial as physical health. The rest of the passage supports this idea.

11. Passage 1: "Climate change is a serious problem that threatens our planet. It is imperative that we take immediate action to reduce our carbon emissions, invest in renewable energy, and conserve our natural resources."

What is the author's primary purpose in this text?
a. To inform the reader about the concept of climate change.
b. To persuade the reader to take action against climate change.
c. To entertain the reader with a story about climate change.
d. To describe the effects of climate change.

Answer: b. To persuade the reader to take action against climate change.
Explanation: The author's main intent in this text is not just to inform the reader about climate change but to persuade them to take immediate action.

12. Passage 2: "The Grand Canyon, located in Arizona, is one of the most popular national parks in the United States. Its deep canyons and colorful cliffs are a sight to behold, attracting millions of tourists each year."

What is the author's primary purpose in this text?
a. To persuade the reader to visit the Grand Canyon.
b. To inform the reader about the Grand Canyon.
c. To entertain the reader with a story about the Grand Canyon.
d. To describe the beauty of the Grand Canyon.

Answer: b. To inform the reader about the Grand Canyon.
Explanation: The author is providing information about the Grand Canyon, making the primary purpose to inform.

13. Passage 3: "Once upon a time, in a land far away, there was a brave knight who set out on a dangerous journey to rescue a princess from a fierce dragon."

What is the author's primary purpose in this text?
a. To inform the reader about the history of knights.
b. To persuade the reader to become a knight.
c. To entertain the reader with a story.
d. To describe the dragon.

Answer: c. To entertain the reader with a story.
Explanation: The classic "Once upon a time" opening suggests a story or tale intended to entertain.

14. Passage 4: "Regular exercise has been proven to have numerous health benefits. It can help control your weight, reduce your risk of heart diseases, and improve your mental health and mood. With all these benefits, there's no reason not to start exercising today."

What is the author's primary purpose in this text?
a. To inform the reader about the benefits of exercise.
b. To persuade the reader to start exercising.
c. To entertain the reader with a story about exercise.
d. To describe different types of exercises.

Answer: b. To persuade the reader to start exercising.

Passage:

The world is fascinated with the concept of time travel, the idea of moving between different points in time. Science fiction authors often depict it in their books, and filmmakers bring it to life on the big screen. But could time travel ever be more than just a figment of our imagination? Could it become a reality?

Albert Einstein's theories of relativity suggest that time travel could indeed be possible, given the right circumstances. In his theories, Einstein explains that time and space are interconnected in what he describes as a four-dimensional fabric called "space-time". The mass of a large object, like a planet, causes a distortion in this fabric, which we experience as gravity. Thus, theoretically, it is possible that an object of sufficient mass and density could distort time itself.

Einstein's theory also postulates that the speed of light is the same for all observers, regardless of their motion or that of the light source. This led to his famous conclusion that time could be slowed down by traveling at very high speeds, a concept often referred to as "time dilation."

Imagine a spacecraft leaving Earth at a speed close to the speed of light, while another identical one stays on Earth. According to Einstein's theory, if these two spacecrafts could communicate with each other, the one in space would perceive time as moving slower than the one on Earth. So, if it were possible to travel at the speed of light, one could theoretically go to the future.

While Einstein's theories provide us with the theoretical foundation for time travel, practical time travel remains a challenge. Traveling at the speed of light or creating an object of sufficient mass to distort time are feats currently beyond our technological capabilities. For now, time travel remains firmly in the realm of science fiction. But who knows what the future holds?

Question:

15. What is the primary focus of this passage?
a. The life and achievements of Albert Einstein
b. The concept of time travel and its theoretical possibilities
c. The process of writing science fiction
d. The development of technologies for space travel

Answer: b. The concept of time travel and its theoretical possibilities
Explanation:The passage primarily discusses the concept of time travel, its representation in popular culture, and its theoretical possibilities as suggested by Einstein's theories of relativity. While the passage does mention Einstein, science fiction, and space travel, these are not its main focus.

Passage:

Over centuries, astronomers have devoted themselves to exploring the mysteries of the universe, and they've made some remarkable discoveries. One of the most fascinating celestial objects they've uncovered is the black hole.

Black holes, so named because even light can't escape their gravitational pull, making them invisible to the naked eye, are formed when a massive star collapses under its own weight. This collapse leads to a singularity, a point of infinite density that warps the fabric of space-time around it. As a result, anything that gets too close to a black hole gets sucked in, including light, hence their name.

The edge of a black hole, where light can't escape, is called the event horizon. This is a point of no return for any object that gets too close. Interestingly, time slows down near a black hole due to the immense gravity, a phenomenon known as time dilation. The idea of wormholes, hypothetical tunnels through space-time, has also been associated with black holes, sparking many scientific debates and inspiring countless works of science fiction.

Although black holes can't be observed directly, astronomers have discovered several methods to detect them, including the observation of high-energy light forms and the effects of gravitational waves. Despite their ominous name and nature, black holes are fascinating objects that continue to captivate scientists and laymen alike.

16. What causes the formation of a black hole?
a. A massive star exploding
b. A massive star collapsing under its own weight
c. A wormhole opening
d. Light escaping from a singularity

Answer: b. A massive star collapsing under its own weight
Explanation: The passage states that black holes are formed when a massive star collapses under its own weight.

17. Why are black holes invisible to the naked eye?
a. They emit high-energy light forms
b. They warp the fabric of space-time
c. Light can't escape their gravitational pull
d. They are actually visible, but very far away

Answer: c. Light can't escape their gravitational pull
Explanation: The passage mentions that even light can't escape the gravitational pull of black holes, making them invisible.

18. What is the event horizon of a black hole?
a. The center of the black hole
b. The point where the black hole starts
c. The edge of the black hole from where light can't escape
d. The point at which the star collapses

Answer: c. The edge of the black hole from where light can't escape
Explanation: The passage defines the event horizon as the edge of a black hole, where light can't escape.

19. What is time dilation in the context of black holes?
a. Time speeds up near a black hole
b. Time stops near a black hole
c. Time slows down near a black hole
d. Time reverses near a black hole

Answer: c. Time slows down near a black hole
Explanation: The passage explains that time slows down near a black hole due to its immense gravity.

20. What is a wormhole as related to black holes?
a. Another name for black holes
b. The center of a black hole
c. Hypothetical tunnels through space-time
d. The path light takes around a black hole

Answer: c. Hypothetical tunnels through space-time
Explanation: The passage describes wormholes as hypothetical tunnels through space-time, associated with black holes.

21. How can black holes be detected?
a. Through direct observation with the naked eye
b. By observing the effects of gravitational waves and high-energy light forms
c. By observing the collapsed stars
d. Through the use of specialized telescopes

Answer: b. By observing the effects of gravitational waves and high-energy light forms
Explanation: The passage states that black holes can be detected through observation of high-energy light forms and the effects of gravitational waves.

22. Which of the following best describes the public interest in black holes?
a. Black holes are largely ignored by the public.
b. Black holes are a subject of fascination and captivation.
c. The public fears black holes due to their ominous nature.
d. Only scientists are interested in black holes.

Answer: b. Black holes are a subject of fascination and captivation.
Explanation: The passage concludes by stating that black holes continue to captivate scientists and laymen alike.

23. What is a singularity in the context of black holes?
a. The collapsed star
b. The event horizon
c. A point of infinite density that warps space-time
d. The high-energy light form emitted by a black hole

Answer: c. A point of infinite density that warps space-time
Explanation: The passage describes a singularity as a point of infinite density that warps the fabric of space-time around it.

24. What happens to objects that get too close to a black hole?
a. They get repelled due to high energy
b. They orbit the black hole
c. They get sucked into the black hole
d. They disappear

Answer: c. They get sucked into the black hole
Explanation: The passage states that anything that gets too close to a black hole gets sucked in, including light.

25. What connection does the passage draw between black holes and science fiction?
a. Science fiction often misrepresents black holes.
b. Black holes have inspired many works of science fiction.
c. Science fiction has contributed to the scientific understanding of black holes.
d. There is no connection between black holes and science fiction.

Answer: b. Black holes have inspired many works of science fiction.
Explanation: The passage notes that the idea of wormholes, associated with black holes, has inspired countless works of science fiction.

Passage:

The rainforests, often referred to as the lungs of the Earth, are unique and diverse ecosystems that are vital for the health of our planet. These vast, dense forests are teeming with life, home to millions of different species, many of which are not found anywhere else.

Rainforests are the world's oldest living ecosystems, with some surviving in their present form for at least 70 million years. They are incredibly diverse and dynamic, containing over half of the world's plant and animal species. A single hectare of rainforest can contain 750 species of trees and 1500 species of higher plants.

However, rainforests are under threat. Deforestation is a significant concern, primarily driven by logging, agriculture, mining, and urban expansion. The resulting loss of habitat can have devastating effects on the wildlife living there and contribute to the extinction of species.

Rainforests also play a crucial role in the global climate. They absorb vast amounts of carbon dioxide, a greenhouse gas that contributes to global warming, and produce about 20% of the world's oxygen. The destruction of these forests not only leads to loss of biodiversity but also exacerbates climate change.

Preserving the rainforests is thus essential for maintaining global biodiversity and combating climate change. Conservation efforts include sustainable logging, the creation of protected areas, and promoting sustainable agriculture practices. With concerted global action, it is possible to preserve these vital ecosystems for future generations.

26. Why are rainforests often referred to as the lungs of the Earth?
a. Because they contain a lot of water
b. Because they absorb carbon dioxide and produce oxygen
c. Because they are the oldest ecosystems on Earth
d. Because they are home to many species

Answer: b. Because they absorb carbon dioxide and produce oxygen
Explanation: The passage mentions that rainforests absorb carbon dioxide, a greenhouse gas, and produce about 20% of the world's oxygen, earning them the nickname "the lungs of the Earth."

27. How many species of trees can a single hectare of rainforest contain?
a. 1500
b. 750
c. 500
d. 1000

Answer: b. 750
Explanation: The passage states that a single hectare of rainforest can contain 750 species of trees.

28. What are the primary drivers of deforestation in rainforests?
a. Logging, agriculture, mining, and urban expansion
b. Natural disasters and climate change
c. Invasive species and disease
d. Tourism and hunting

Answer: a. Logging, agriculture, mining, and urban expansion
Explanation: The passage identifies logging, agriculture, mining, and urban expansion as significant contributors to deforestation in rainforests.

29. What does the loss of rainforests contribute to?
a. Improved air quality
b. Reduction in global warming
c. Extinction of species and climate change
d. Increase in biodiversity

Answer: c. Extinction of species and climate change
Explanation: The passage explains that the destruction of rainforests can lead to the extinction of species and exacerbate climate change.

30. What are some of the conservation efforts mentioned in the passage?
a. Creating wildlife reserves and banning logging
b. Sustainable logging, creating protected areas, and promoting sustainable agriculture practices
c. Relocating wildlife and reintroducing extinct species
d. Planting more trees and reducing carbon emissions

Answer: b. Sustainable logging, creating protected areas, and promoting sustainable agriculture practices
Explanation: The passage mentions sustainable logging, the creation of protected areas, and promoting sustainable agriculture practices as methods of conserving rainforests.

31. What percentage of the world's oxygen is produced by rainforests?
a. 10%
b. 20%
c. 30%
d. 50%

Answer: b. 20%
Explanation: The passage mentions that rainforests produce about 20% of the world's oxygen.

32. Why is the destruction of rainforests a concern for global climate?
a. Because it reduces the amount of oxygen produced
b. Because it exacerbates global warming
c. Because it disrupts the water cycle
d. Because it increases carbon dioxide levels

Answer: b. Because it exacerbates global warming
Explanation: The passage mentions that the destruction of rainforests exacerbates global warming, as these forests absorb vast amounts of carbon dioxide, a greenhouse gas.

33. How many species of higher plants can a single hectare of rainforest contain?
a. 500
b. 750
c. 1000
d. 1500

Answer: d. 1500. Explanation: The passage states that a single hectare of rainforest can contain 1500 species of higher plants.

34. Why is preserving rainforests essential?
a. For tourism and recreation
b. For maintaining global biodiversity and combating climate change
c. For scientific research
d. For economic reasons

Answer: b. For maintaining global biodiversity and combating climate change
Explanation: The passage states that preserving the rainforests is crucial for maintaining global biodiversity and combating climate change.

35. How old are the world's oldest living rainforest ecosystems?
a. 1 million years
b. 10 million years
c. 50 million years
d. 70 million years

Answer: d. 70 million years
Explanation: The passage says that the world's oldest living rainforest ecosystems have survived in their present form for at least 70 million years.

Passage:

The exploration of space has been a key part of human advancement. Starting with the launch of the Soviet satellite Sputnik in 1957, we have been continuously reaching for the stars. In 1969, the United States achieved the monumental feat of landing the first humans on the moon. The Apollo missions continued until 1972, bringing back valuable lunar rock samples. Meanwhile, unmanned missions have been sent to all the planets in the solar system, providing us with detailed information about our planetary neighbors.

36. What was the name of the first satellite launched into space?
a. Explorer
b. Apollo
c. Sputnik
d. Voyager

Answer: c. Sputnik

37. Which country landed the first humans on the moon?
a. United States
b. Russia
c. China
d. India

Answer: a. United States

38. When did the first moon landing occur?
a. 1961
b. 1969
c. 1972
d. 1979

Answer: b. 1969

39. What did the Apollo missions bring back from the moon?
a. Lunar rock samples
b. Alien artifacts
c. Water ice
d. Solar wind particles

Answer: a. Lunar rock samples

40. Which planet has not been reached by an unmanned mission?
a. Venus
b. Jupiter
c. Uranus
d. None of the above

Answer: d. None of the above

41. What was the purpose of the Apollo missions?
a. To establish a base on the moon
b. To test the limits of human endurance
c. To bring back samples from the moon
d. To prepare for a mission to Mars

Answer: c. To bring back samples from the moon

42. What was the first major accomplishment in space exploration?
a. Man walking on the moon
b. Launching a satellite into space
c. Sending a rover to Mars
d. Photographing a black hole

Answer: b. Launching a satellite into space

43. Who launched the Sputnik satellite?
a. United States
b. Russia (Soviet Union)
c. European Space Agency
d. China

Answer: b. Russia (Soviet Union)

44. What information have unmanned missions provided us with?
a. Detailed information about our planetary neighbors
b. A map of the entire universe
c. The existence of extraterrestrial life
d. A way to communicate with aliens

Answer: a. Detailed information about our planetary neighbors

45. What year did the Apollo missions end?
a. 1969
b. 1970
c. 1972
d. 1975

Answer: c. 1972

Passage:

The Amazon rainforest, spanning over 2.1 million square miles, is one of the most biodiverse regions on the planet, home to an estimated 400 billion individual trees from 16,000 species. Often referred to as the "lungs of the Earth," the Amazon rainforest produces around 20% of the world's oxygen. However, this ecological treasure is under threat due to extensive deforestation and climate change.

Deforestation in the Amazon is mainly driven by human activities such as agriculture, logging, and infrastructure development. Agricultural activities, especially cattle ranching and soy production, are responsible for about 80% of deforestation. As trees are cut down, the carbon they have stored is released into the atmosphere, leading to increased levels of carbon dioxide, a key contributor to global warming.

Efforts to curb deforestation include the implementation of strict logging laws and the promotion of sustainable farming practices. In addition, several international initiatives aim to protect the Amazon rainforest by providing financial incentives to countries and communities to conserve forests and invest in low-carbon development paths. Despite these efforts, the rate of deforestation in the Amazon is still alarming, and more urgent actions are needed to preserve this vital ecosystem.

46. What is the Amazon rainforest often referred to as?
a. The heart of the Earth
b. The lungs of the Earth
c. The brain of the Earth
d. The veins of the Earth

Answer: b. The lungs of the Earth

47. What percentage of the world's oxygen does the Amazon rainforest produce?
a. 10%
b. 20%
c. 30%
d. 40%

Answer: b. 20%

48. What is the main driver of deforestation in the Amazon?
a. Natural disasters
b. Human activities
c. Climate change
d. Animal activities

Answer: b. Human activities

49. What agricultural activities are largely responsible for deforestation in the Amazon?
a. Rice cultivation and poultry farming
b. Cattle ranching and soy production
c. Wheat farming and dairy production
d. Corn farming and pig farming

Answer: b. Cattle ranching and soy production

50. What happens when trees are cut down in the Amazon rainforest?
a. The soil becomes more fertile
b. The level of carbon dioxide decreases
c. The stored carbon is released, contributing to global warming
d. The rate of photosynthesis increases

Answer: c. The stored carbon is released, contributing to global warming

51. What are the efforts to curb deforestation in the Amazon?
a. Building more infrastructure
b. Implementing strict logging laws and promoting sustainable farming
c. Encouraging agricultural expansion
d. Investing in high-carbon development paths

Answer: b. Implementing strict logging laws and promoting sustainable farming

52. How do international initiatives aim to protect the Amazon rainforest?
a. By providing financial incentives to conserve forests and invest in low-carbon development paths
b. By promoting the use of fossil fuels
c. By encouraging more logging activities
d. By supporting large-scale agriculture

Answer: a. By providing financial incentives to conserve forests and invest in low-carbon development paths

53. What is the current state of deforestation in the Amazon?
a. It has completely stopped
b. It has significantly reduced
c. It is increasing at an alarming rate
d. It is fluctuating but stable

Answer: c. It is increasing at an alarming rate

54. What is the estimated number of individual trees in the Amazon rainforest?
a. 400 million
b. 400 billion
c. 4 trillion
d. 4 quadrillion

Answer: b. 400 billion

55. How many tree species are estimated to be in the Amazon rainforest?
a. 1,600
b. 16,000
c. 160,000
d. 1.6 million

Answer: b. 16,000

Passage:

The Great Pyramid of Giza, built as a tomb for the Egyptian pharaoh Khufu, is one of the Seven Wonders of the Ancient World and the only one to remain largely intact. Constructed around 2560 BC, it was the tallest man-made structure for over 3,800 years, standing at a staggering 146.6 meters (481 feet).

The pyramid was built using approximately 2.3 million blocks of stone, each weighing an average of 2.5 tons. Its construction is still a subject of debate among researchers. The most widely accepted theory is that it was built using a system of ramps to move the blocks into place.

The Great Pyramid has three known chambers: the King's Chamber, the Queen's Chamber, and the Unfinished Chamber. The King's Chamber contains a granite sarcophagus, which is believed to have held the body of Pharaoh Khufu.

Despite the pyramid's age, new discoveries are still being made. In 2017, scientists used muon radiography to detect a previously unknown void inside the pyramid, adding another layer of mystery to this ancient marvel.

56. Who was the Great Pyramid of Giza built for?
a. Pharaoh Ramses
b. Pharaoh Khufu
c. Pharaoh Tutankhamun
d. Pharaoh Nefertiti

Answer: b. Pharaoh Khufu

57. When was the Great Pyramid of Giza constructed?
a. Around 3560 BC
b. Around 2560 BC
c. Around 1560 BC
d. Around 560 BC

Answer: b. Around 2560 BC

58. What is the height of the Great Pyramid of Giza?
a. 346.6 meters
b. 246.6 meters
c. 146.6 meters
d. 46.6 meters

Answer: c. 146.6 meters

59. How many blocks of stone were used in the construction of the Great Pyramid?
a. 230,000
b. 2.3 million
c. 23 million
d. 230 million

Answer: b. 2.3 million

60. What was the average weight of the stone blocks used in the construction of the pyramid?
a. 0.5 tons
b. 1.5 tons
c. 2.5 tons
d. 3.5 tons

Answer: c. 2.5 tons

61. What does the King's Chamber in the pyramid contain?
a. Gold treasures
b. Hieroglyphic inscriptions
c. A granite sarcophagus
d. A large statue of Khufu

Answer: c. A granite sarcophagus

62. What is the most widely accepted theory about how the pyramid was built?
a. Using a system of pulleys
b. Using a system of ramps
c. Using alien technology
d. Using a large workforce of slaves

Answer: b. Using a system of ramps

63. What is the Great Pyramid of Giza known as?
a. One of the Seven Wonders of the Modern World
b. One of the Seven Wonders of the Ancient World
c. One of the Seven Wonders of Egypt
d. One of the Seven Wonders of Africa

Answer: b. One of the Seven Wonders of the Ancient World

64. What recent discovery was made inside the Great Pyramid?
a. A new treasure room
b. An unknown void
c. A hidden tomb
d. A secret passage

Answer: b. An unknown void

65. How long was the Great Pyramid the tallest man-made structure?
a. Over 2,800 years
b. Over 3,800 years
c. Over 4,800 years
d. Over 5,800 years

Answer: b. Over 3,800 years

Passage: The Amazon Rainforest, often referred to as the "lungs of the Earth", is the world's largest tropical rainforest. It spans over nine countries in South America, with the majority of it located in Brazil. It is home to an estimated 400 billion individual trees representing 16,000 species and a wide array of diverse wildlife, some of which are not found anywhere else on the planet.

The Amazon Rainforest plays a crucial role in the global climate. It absorbs vast quantities of carbon dioxide, a greenhouse gas that contributes to global warming, and produces about 20% of the world's oxygen. However, this important ecosystem is under threat due to deforestation, largely driven by logging, mining, and agricultural activities.

Several Indigenous tribes also inhabit the Amazon, living in harmony with nature for thousands of years. Their knowledge of the forest's flora and fauna is invaluable for conservation efforts and scientific research.

In recent years, there has been a global call to protect the Amazon Rainforest. Multiple non-profit organizations, governments, and even corporations are collaborating to halt its destruction and restore the lost areas.

66. What is the Amazon Rainforest often referred to as?
a. Heart of the Earth
b. Lungs of the Earth
c. Brain of the Earth
d. Kidneys of the Earth

Answer: b. Lungs of the Earth

67. How many countries does the Amazon Rainforest span over?
a. Six
b. Seven
c. Eight
d. Nine

Answer: d. Nine

68. What percentage of the world's oxygen is produced by the Amazon Rainforest?
a. 10%
b. 20%
c. 30%
d. 40%

Answer: b. 20%

69. What is the major cause of deforestation in the Amazon Rainforest?
a. Logging, mining, and agriculture
b. Natural disasters
c. Urbanization
d. Climate change

Answer: a. Logging, mining, and agriculture

70. Who has lived in harmony with nature in the Amazon Rainforest for thousands of years?
a. Local farmers
b. Indigenous tribes
c. Wildlife researchers
d. Government officials

Answer: b. Indigenous tribes

71. What is a crucial role of the Amazon Rainforest in the global climate?
a. It absorbs a vast amount of carbon dioxide.
b. It produces a high quantity of carbon dioxide.
c. It reduces the earth's temperature.
d. It increases rainfall in the region.

Answer: a. It absorbs a vast amount of carbon dioxide.

72. Which country has the majority of the Amazon Rainforest?
a. Peru
b. Colombia
c. Venezuela
d. Brazil

Answer: d. Brazil

73. What is the approximate number of individual trees in the Amazon Rainforest?
a. 400 million
b. 400 billion
c. 4 trillion
d. 40 trillion

Answer: b. 400 billion

74. How many species of trees are estimated to be in the Amazon Rainforest?
a. 1,600
b. 16,000
c. 160,000
d. 1,600,000

Answer: b. 16,000

75. What recent global initiative is taking place regarding the Amazon Rainforest?
a. Ignoring its importance
b. Exploiting its resources
c. Protecting and restoring it
d. Converting it into agricultural land

Answer: c. Protecting and restoring it

Passage: The sport of basketball has come a long way since its inception. Invented by Dr. James Naismith in 1891, basketball began as a simple game with a soccer ball and two peach baskets. Naismith wrote down 13 basic rules, many of which are still in effect in some form today.

The National Basketball Association (NBA) was established in 1946. The NBA quickly became the premier professional basketball league in the world, a title it still holds. The NBA was also revolutionary in its inclusion of African American athletes, changing the face of professional sports in the United States.

Over the years, basketball has transformed, with rule changes, new technology, and the influence of legendary players. Figures like Michael Jordan, Magic Johnson, and Kobe Bryant have become household names, inspiring new generations of players and fans alike.

Today, basketball is a global phenomenon, with the NBA's influence reaching far beyond the United States. The sport is played professionally in many countries, and international players have become NBA stars. Basketball's popularity continues to grow, bridging cultural divides and uniting people around a shared love of the game.

76. Who invented basketball?
a. Michael Jordan
b. Dr. James Naismith
c. Magic Johnson
d. Kobe Bryant

Answer: b. Dr. James Naismith

77. When was the NBA established?
a. 1891
b. 1946
c. 1961
d. 1986

Answer: b. 1946

78. Which of the following best summarizes paragraph 2?
a. The NBA was established in 1946 and quickly became the leading professional basketball league globally.
b. Dr. James Naismith invented basketball in 1891.
c. Basketball has evolved through rule changes, new technology, and influential players.
d. Basketball is a worldwide phenomenon with professional leagues in many countries.

Answer: a. The NBA was established in 1946 and quickly became the leading professional basketball league globally.

79. What did the NBA change about professional sports in the United States?
a. It introduced basketball as a new sport.
b. It included African American athletes.
c. It started the trend of tall players.
d. It started using peach baskets as goals.

Answer: b. It included African American athletes.

80. Which detail is irrelevant to the main idea of paragraph 4?
a. NBA's influence reaches far beyond the United States.
b. Basketball is played professionally in many countries.
c. International players have become NBA stars.
d. Dr. James Naismith wrote down 13 basic rules.

Answer: d. Dr. James Naismith wrote down 13 basic rules.

81. Who among the following is not mentioned as a legendary player?
a. Michael Jordan
b. Magic Johnson
c. Kobe Bryant
d. LeBron James

Answer: d. LeBron James

82. When was basketball invented?
a. 1891
b. 1946
c. 1961
d. 1986

Answer: a. 1891

83. What was basketball initially played with?
a. A soccer ball and two peach baskets
b. A rugby ball and two nets
c. A leather ball and two hoops
d. A wooden ball and two barrels

Answer: a. A soccer ball and two peach baskets

84. What is the global impact of basketball today?
a. It is only popular in the United States.
b. It is played professionally only in a few countries.
c. It is a global phenomenon and unites people across cultures.
d. It is a fading sport with reducing popularity.

Answer: c. It is a global phenomenon and unites people across cultures.

85. What is an ongoing trend in the sport of basketball?
a. The influence of legendary players is declining.
b. Rule changes and new technology continue to transform the game.
c. The NBA is losing its global influence.
d. Basketball is losing popularity.

Answer: b. Rule changes and new technology continue to transform the game.

Passage:The debate over the value of artificial intelligence (AI) in our society is a fiery one. Proponents argue that AI can streamline processes, increase efficiency, and even lead to novel discoveries in various fields such as medicine and astronomy.

Opponents, however, caution against the overreliance on technology, highlighting potential drawbacks such as job losses and privacy concerns. Furthermore, they point out that artificial intelligence lacks the emotional intelligence and nuanced understanding that human workers provide.

Yet, it's impossible to ignore the significant impact that AI already has on our daily lives. From search engine algorithms that curate personalized internet experiences to voice-activated assistants like Siri and Alexa, artificial intelligence is everywhere. Even in fields like healthcare, AI is making a mark, with machine learning algorithms helping to analyze complex medical data.

As we move further into the digital age, the role of artificial intelligence is only set to expand. Despite the challenges, the potential benefits of AI integration in various sectors are vast. Still, it is crucial that we continue to critically evaluate the implications of this technology on our society and our future.

86. What is the main argument of proponents of AI?
a. AI lacks emotional intelligence.
b. AI can lead to job losses.
c. AI can streamline processes and lead to novel discoveries.
d. AI is a threat to privacy.

Answer: c. AI can streamline processes and lead to novel discoveries.

87. Which of the following best summarizes paragraph 2?
a. AI is increasing efficiency in various fields.
b. Opponents of AI highlight potential drawbacks including job losses and privacy concerns.
c. AI is making a mark in healthcare.
d. AI is expanding its role in the digital age.

Answer: b. Opponents of AI highlight potential drawbacks including job losses and privacy concerns.

88. Which of these is not a current application of AI mentioned in the passage?
a. Analyzing complex medical data.
b. Curating personalized internet experiences.
c. Serving as voice-activated assistants.
d. Driving autonomous vehicles.

Answer: d. Driving autonomous vehicles.

89. What do opponents of AI emphasize?
a. The streamlined processes of AI.
b. The potential drawbacks such as job losses and privacy concerns.
c. The role of AI in the digital age.
d. The presence of AI in daily lives.

Answer: b. The potential drawbacks such as job losses and privacy concerns.

90. Which detail is irrelevant to the main idea of paragraph 4?
a. AI already has a significant impact on our daily lives.
b. Search engine algorithms curate personalized internet experiences.
c. AI is everywhere, including in healthcare.
d. Opponents caution against the overreliance on technology.

Answer: d. Opponents caution against the overreliance on technology.

91. What is the anticipated future of AI according to the passage?
a. AI is expected to decline in the future.
b. The role of AI is only set to expand.
c. AI is expected to replace all human workers.
d. AI will eventually be obsolete.

Answer: b. The role of AI is only set to expand.

92. What is one area where AI has made a mark?
a. Public transportation.
b. Healthcare.
c. Food service.
d. Clothing production.

Answer: b. Healthcare.

93. What does the passage suggest about AI's emotional intelligence?
a. AI has superior emotional intelligence.
b. AI has comparable emotional intelligence to humans.
c. AI lacks the emotional intelligence and nuanced understanding that human workers provide.
d. The emotional intelligence of AI is not mentioned in the passage.

Answer: c. AI lacks the emotional intelligence and nuanced understanding that human workers provide.

94. What is a concern related to the integration of AI in various sectors?
a. Increased efficiency.
b. Novel discoveries.
c. Job losses and privacy concerns.
d. Streamlined processes.

Answer: c. Job losses and privacy concerns.

95. What does the passage suggest should be done regarding the implications of AI?
a. They should be ignored.
b. They should be embraced without question.
c. They should be critically evaluated.
d. They should be dismissed.

Answer: c. They should be critically evaluated.

Passage: In the realm of quantum physics, particles behave in ways that baffle scientists and laymen alike. One such curious phenomenon is quantum entanglement, where two particles become connected so that the state of one can instantly affect the other, no matter the distance.

This quantum connection might seem like something out of a science fiction novel, but it's actually a fundamental aspect of quantum mechanics. The entangled particles could be light-years apart, but the change in the state of one will immediately affect the other. Albert Einstein famously referred to this as "spooky action at a distance."

Despite the baffling nature of quantum entanglement, it holds promising potential for various fields. For instance, it could revolutionize communication technology by enabling faster-than-light data transfer. In cryptography, it could enhance security by alerting users to eavesdroppers, as any interference would immediately change the state of the entangled particles.

However, realizing these applications is challenging due to the fragile nature of quantum entanglement. Any disturbance, such as heat or light, can easily disrupt the quantum state. As such, much of the research in this field is focused on overcoming these challenges and harnessing the potential of quantum entanglement in a practical way.

96. What is the primary concept discussed in the passage?
a. Cryptography.
b. Communication technology.
c. Quantum entanglement.
d. Albert Einstein.

Answer: c. Quantum entanglement.

97. Which of the following best summarizes paragraph 2?
a. Quantum entanglement is a science fiction concept.
b. Quantum entanglement allows for instantaneous connection between particles regardless of distance.
c. Quantum entanglement has been dismissed by Albert Einstein.
d. Quantum entanglement interferes with data transfer.

Answer: b. Quantum entanglement allows for instantaneous connection between particles regardless of distance.

98. What did Albert Einstein refer to quantum entanglement as?
a. A science fiction concept.
b. Spooky action at a distance.
c. An unsolvable mystery.
d. A disruptive phenomenon.

Answer: b. Spooky action at a distance.

99. Which potential application of quantum entanglement is discussed in the passage?
a. Power generation.
b. Faster-than-light data transfer.
c. Space exploration.
d. Medical diagnostics.

Answer: b. Faster-than-light data transfer.

100. Which detail is irrelevant to the main idea of paragraph 3?
a. Quantum entanglement holds promising potential.
b. It could enhance security in cryptography.
c. Any interference would immediately change the state of entangled particles.
d. Albert Einstein referred to this as "spooky action at a distance."

Answer: d. Albert Einstein referred to this as "spooky action at a distance."

101. What is a significant challenge in realizing the potential applications of quantum entanglement?
a. Its confusing nature.
b. Its lack of practicality.
c. Its disruption of communication technology.
d. Its fragility and susceptibility to disturbances.

Answer: d. Its fragility and susceptibility to disturbances.

102. What does the current research in quantum entanglement focus on?
a. Understanding Albert Einstein's perspective.
b. Overcoming challenges and harnessing its potential.
c. Explaining it to laymen.
d. Finding its origin.

Answer: b. Overcoming challenges and harnessing its potential.

103. What is a unique characteristic of quantum entanglement?
a. It enables faster-than-light data transfer.
b. It is easily disrupted by heat and light.
c. The state of one particle can instantly affect the entangled particle, regardless of distance.
d. It is only a theoretical concept.

Answer: c. The state of one particle can instantly affect the entangled particle, regardless of distance.

104. How could quantum entanglement be beneficial in cryptography?
a. It could create unbreakable codes.
b. It could alert users to eavesdroppers.
c. It could decode encrypted messages.
d. It could replace traditional methods.

Answer: b. It could alert users to eavesdroppers.

105. What is the main idea of the passage?
a. Quantum entanglement is a confusing concept.
b. Quantum entanglement could revolutionize various fields but is challenging to apply.
c. Albert Einstein disapproved of quantum entanglement.
d. Quantum entanglement is disrupting communication technology.

Answer: b. Quantum entanglement could revolutionize various fields but is challenging to apply.

Passage:Often touted as one of the world's most resilient creatures, the tardigrade, or water bear, continues to amaze scientists with its survival capabilities. These micro-animals, measuring less than a millimeter long, are found in diverse habitats around the globe, from the highest mountains to the deepest oceans.

Tardigrades can withstand extreme conditions that would be fatal to most other life forms. They have been observed to survive temperatures as low as -272.8 degrees Celsius and as high as 150 degrees Celsius. Moreover, tardigrades can tolerate pressures six times greater than those found in the deepest ocean trenches, and can survive in the vacuum of outer space.

These extraordinary survival skills are attributed to a process called cryptobiosis. When faced with adverse conditions, a tardigrade's metabolism slows down drastically, entering a state of suspended animation where all metabolic processes stop. In this state, they can endure for years or even decades until conditions become favorable again.

Researchers hope that by understanding more about the tardigrade's survival mechanisms, we can develop new techniques to protect human cells. For instance, during space travel, human cells could potentially be made more resistant to radiation damage.

106. What creature is primarily discussed in this passage?
a. Humans
b. Mountain animals
c. Tardigrades
d. Deep sea creatures

Answer: c. Tardigrades

107. Which of the following best summarizes paragraph 2?
a. Tardigrades are fatal to most other life forms.
b. Tardigrades can survive in extreme conditions, including very high and low temperatures, great pressure, and the vacuum of outer space.
c. Tardigrades prefer to live in cold, high-pressure environments.
d. Tardigrades have been sent to outer space for research purposes.

Answer: b. Tardigrades can survive in extreme conditions, including very high and low temperatures, great pressure, and the vacuum of outer space.

108. What is cryptobiosis?
a. A type of habitat for tardigrades.
b. A survival technique where tardigrades enter a state of suspended animation.
c. The process of tardigrades growing larger.
d. The ability of tardigrades to live in outer space.

Answer: b. A survival technique where tardigrades enter a state of suspended animation.

109. Which detail is irrelevant to the main idea of paragraph 3?
a. Cryptobiosis is a process that slows down a tardigrade's metabolism.
b. Tardigrades can endure for years or even decades in a state of cryptobiosis.
c. All metabolic processes stop in a tardigrade during cryptobiosis.
d. Tardigrades are found in diverse habitats around the globe.

Answer: d. Tardigrades are found in diverse habitats around the globe.

110. How might understanding tardigrades' survival mechanisms benefit humans?
a. It could help humans survive in the vacuum of outer space.
b. It could help develop new techniques to protect human cells.
c. It could help humans survive extreme temperatures.
d. It could help humans live in diverse habitats.

Answer: b. It could help develop new techniques to protect human cells.

111. What is a unique ability of tardigrades mentioned in the passage?
a. Ability to change color.
b. Ability to live in diverse habitats.
c. Ability to survive in the vacuum of outer space.
d. Ability to live underwater.

Answer: c. Ability to survive in the vacuum of outer space.

112. How do tardigrades survive adverse conditions?
a. They move to a safer location.
b. They enter a state of cryptobiosis.
c. They alter their body shape.
d. They reproduce rapidly.

Answer: b. They enter a state of cryptobiosis.

113 Which of the following can tardigrades tolerate?
a. Only high temperatures.
b. Only low temperatures.
c. Neither high nor low temperatures.
d. Both high and low temperatures.

Answer: d. Both high and low temperatures.

114. What is the main idea of the passage?
a. Tardigrades are small creatures that can be found everywhere.
b. Tardigrades are unique creatures that can survive extreme conditions due to their ability to enter a state of cryptobiosis.
c. Tardigrades live in outer space.
d. Tardigrades are a threat to other life forms.

Answer: b. Tardigrades are unique creatures that can survive extreme conditions due to their ability to enter a state of cryptobiosis.

115. What potential benefit does research on tardigrades offer to human space travel?
a. It could make human cells more resistant to radiation damage.
b. It could help humans enter a state of cryptobiosis.
c. It could allow humans to survive in the vacuum of space.
d. It could increase human endurance to high and low temperatures.

Answer: a. It could make human cells more resistant to radiation damage.

Passage: The origin of pasta is a topic of debate amongst food historians. While some posit that the concept was brought to Italy from China by Marco Polo in the 13th century, evidence suggests that pasta was being produced in Italy long before Polo's travels. The Sicilian Arabs in the 9th century were known to have a food of flour in the shape of strings.

In terms of the industrial production of pasta, it was initially made at home, with families having their own traditional shapes and recipes. The industrial production of pasta did not occur until the 19th century when factory systems started to emerge. By the late 19th century, the pasta industry flourished in Italy, especially in the city of Naples.

Pasta has since become a staple food in many countries, especially in Italy, due to its versatility and ease of preparation. It can be served with a wide variety of sauces, meats, vegetables, and cheese. In fact, there are over 600 different shapes of pasta, each designed to hold a specific type of sauce.

Despite its complex history, one thing remains clear: pasta is beloved by people all over the world. Its infinite possibilities for flavor combinations and its comforting, filling nature make it a popular choice for both home cooks and professional chefs.

116. What food is primarily discussed in this passage?
a. Pizza
b. Sushi
c. Pasta
d. Rice

Answer: c. Pasta

117. Which of the following best summarizes paragraph 2?
a. Pasta was traditionally made at home before the industrial production started in the 19th century.
b. Pasta was not popular until the 19th century.
c. Pasta is only produced industrially now.
d. All families have their own traditional pasta shapes and recipes.

Answer: a. Pasta was traditionally made at home before the industrial production started in the 19th century.

118. How many shapes of pasta are mentioned in the passage?
a. Over 500
b. Over 600
c. Over 700
d. Over 800

Answer: b. Over 600

119. Which detail is irrelevant to the main idea of paragraph 3?
a. Pasta is a staple food in many countries.
b. Pasta can be served with a wide variety of accompaniments.
c. There are over 600 different shapes of pasta.
d. The origin of pasta is a topic of debate amongst food historians.

Answer: d. The origin of pasta is a topic of debate amongst food historians.

120. Where did the industrial production of pasta flourish in the late 19th century?
a. Rome
b. Sicily
c. Naples
d. Milan

Answer: c. Naples

121. What is a unique characteristic of pasta mentioned in the passage?
a. Its affordability
b. Its ability to be paired with a variety of sauces, meats, vegetables, and cheese.
c. Its sweet taste
d. Its origin in China

Answer: b. Its ability to be paired with a variety of sauces, meats, vegetables, and cheese.

122. What is the main idea of the last paragraph?
a. Pasta has a complex history.
b. Pasta is beloved by people all over the world due to its versatility and comforting nature.
c. Pasta is a popular choice for professional chefs.
d. The flavor combinations of pasta are infinite.

Answer: b. Pasta is beloved by people all over the world due to its versatility and comforting nature.

123. What evidence suggests that pasta was not brought to Italy by Marco Polo?
a. Pasta was being produced in Italy before Marco Polo's travels.
b. Pasta was a common food in the 13th century.
c. Pasta was introduced to Italy by the Sicilian Arabs.
d. Marco Polo never went to China.

Answer: a. Pasta was being produced in Italy before Marco Polo's travels.

124. What is one reason for pasta's popularity in Italy?
a. It is only made in Italy.
b. It is cheap and easy to prepare.
c. It is usually served with rice.
d. It is exported from Italy to China.

Answer: b. It is cheap and easy to prepare.

125. What does the passage suggest about the traditional preparation of pasta?
a. It was initially made industrially.
b. It was made at home with families having their own traditional shapes and recipes.
c. It was made with a wide variety of sauces, meats, vegetables, and cheese.
d. It was not made until the late 19th century.

Answer: b. It was made at home with families having their own traditional shapes and recipes.

Passage: In a world increasingly driven by technology, the importance of computer science education cannot be overstated. Schools and universities across the globe are now integrating computer science in their curriculum, starting as early as elementary school. It's not just about creating the next generation of software engineers but about equipping students with essential skills for the digital age.

Understanding computer science opens a world of opportunities. Not only does it lead to high-paying jobs, but it also fosters problem-solving skills, logical thinking, and creativity. A basic knowledge of coding, for example, is now regarded as a crucial skill, similar to reading, writing, and arithmetic. Some even consider it as the 'fourth literacy'.

Furthermore, technology plays a crucial role in many sectors, including healthcare, finance, education, and more. For instance, the healthcare industry greatly benefits from advancements in medical technology, such as telemedicine, health informatics, and even robotic surgery.

However, the integration of computer science into the education system is not without challenges. The rapid advancement of technology requires constant updating of the curriculum, which can be a significant task for educators. Additionally, there's a need for qualified teachers who not only understand computer science but can also effectively communicate its complexities to students.

Despite these challenges, the consensus among educators and industry experts is clear: computer science education is not a luxury but a necessity in the 21st century. Its benefits far outweigh its challenges, and every effort should be made to ensure all students have access to this vital field of study.

126. What is the primary focus of this passage?
a. The integration of computer science into education
b. The rapid advancement of technology
c. The challenges faced by educators
d. The importance of telemedicine in healthcare

Answer: a. The integration of computer science into education

127. Which of the following best summarizes paragraph 2?
a. Understanding computer science opens many job opportunities and fosters important skills.
b. A basic knowledge of coding is now regarded as the 'fourth literacy'.
c. Computer science is only about creating software engineers.
d. Creativity is not important in computer science.

Answer: a. Understanding computer science opens many job opportunities and fosters important skills.

128. What industry is mentioned as benefiting from advancements in technology?
a. Fashion
b. Healthcare
c. Automobile
d. Agriculture

Answer: b. Healthcare

129. Which detail is irrelevant to the main idea of paragraph 4?
a. The integration of computer science into the education system faces challenges.
b. The rapid advancement of technology requires constant updating of the curriculum.
c. There's a need for qualified teachers who can effectively communicate computer science to students.
d. The healthcare industry greatly benefits from advancements in medical technology.

Answer: d. The healthcare industry greatly benefits from advancements in medical technology.

130. What is described as the 'fourth literacy' in the passage?
a. Logical thinking
b. Creativity
c. Coding
d. Problem-solving

Answer: c. Coding

131. What is the main idea of the final paragraph?
a. Computer science education is a luxury.
b. Computer science education is a necessity and its benefits far outweigh its challenges.
c. Only a few students should have access to computer science education.
d. Industry experts disagree about the importance of computer science education.

Answer: b. Computer science education is a necessity and its benefits far outweigh its challenges.

132. According to the passage, why is computer science education important?
a. It helps students become software engineers.
b. It fosters problem-solving skills, logical thinking, and creativity.
c. It allows students to understand telemedicine.
d. It is only important for high-paying jobs.

Answer: b. It fosters problem-solving skills, logical thinking, and creativity.

133. What is the main challenge in integrating computer science into the education system, as per the passage?
a. The need for high-paying jobs
b. The rapid advancement of technology requires constant updating of the curriculum.
c. Lack of interest among students
d. Lack of computer systems in schools

Answer: b. The rapid advancement of technology requires constant updating of the curriculum.

134. What is the consensus among educators and industry experts regarding computer science education?
a. It is not important.
b. It is a necessity in the 21st century.
c. It should be taught only at university level.
d. It is only for students interested in software engineering.

Answer: b. It is a necessity in the 21st century.

135. Which paragraph provides specific examples of how technology plays a crucial role in various sectors?
a. Paragraph 1
b. Paragraph 2
c. Paragraph 3
d. Paragraph 4

Answer: c. Paragraph 3

Passage: Water is a fundamental resource, underpinning all aspects of human and ecological existence. Yet, the world is facing a water crisis that is not only environmental but also social and political. Lack of access to clean, safe water is a pervasive problem, impacting billions of people worldwide. It exacerbates poverty, creates health issues, and can even trigger conflicts and migration.

The water crisis is particularly acute in developing countries, where infrastructure for water management is often inadequate. However, even in developed nations, water scarcity can be a serious issue due to pollution, overuse, and climate change effects such as droughts. For instance, Cape Town in South Africa, once faced a significant threat of running out of water, a phenomenon known as 'Day Zero'.

Efforts to address this crisis must focus not just on increasing water supply but also on improving water quality and promoting sustainable water management. This includes measures such as reducing water waste, reusing water where possible, and protecting water sources from pollution.

Technological innovation also plays a crucial role. From simple, low-cost filtration devices that can provide clean water in remote areas, to large-scale desalination plants that can convert seawater into freshwater, technology offers potential solutions.

However, addressing the water crisis requires more than just technological solutions. It demands political will, effective policies, and international cooperation. Equitable access to water must be recognized as a human right and protected as such, a challenge that will require collective action and substantial effort.

136. What is the primary concern addressed in this passage?
a. The importance of technological innovation
b. The issue of water scarcity and its implications
c. The effects of climate change
d. The lack of political will to address crises

Answer: b. The issue of water scarcity and its implications

137. Which of the following best summarizes paragraph 2?
a. Developing countries are solely responsible for the water crisis.
b. Both developing and developed countries experience water scarcity due to various factors.
c. Cape Town has already run out of water.
d. Developed nations do not face water scarcity.

Answer: b. Both developing and developed countries experience water scarcity due to various factors.

138. What are some measures suggested for sustainable water management in the passage?
a. Increasing water supply only
b. Reducing water waste, reusing water, and protecting water sources from pollution
c. Building large-scale desalination plants only
d. Ignoring water quality

Answer: b. Reducing water waste, reusing water, and protecting water sources from pollution

139. Which detail is irrelevant to the main idea of paragraph 4?
a. Technological innovation plays a crucial role in addressing the water crisis.
b. Filtration devices can provide clean water in remote areas.
c. Desalination plants can convert seawater into freshwater.
d. Equitable access to water must be recognized as a human right.

Answer: d. Equitable access to water must be recognized as a human right.

140. What is referred to as 'Day Zero' in the passage?
a. The day when water quality improves
b. The day when a city runs out of water
c. The day when water management becomes sustainable
d. The day when the water crisis is solved

Answer: b. The day when a city runs out of water

141. According to the passage, what besides technological solutions is needed to address the water crisis?
a. Ignoring the crisis
b. Political will, effective policies, and international cooperation
c. Sole reliance on desalination plants
d. Not recognizing water access as a human right

Answer: b. Political will, effective policies, and international cooperation

142. What is the main idea of the final paragraph?
a. Technological solutions are sufficient to address the water crisis.
b. Equitable access to water should be recognized as a human right, requiring collective action and substantial effort.
c. The water crisis is solely a political issue.
d. Water quality is irrelevant to the water crisis.

Answer: b. Equitable access to water should be recognized as a human right, requiring collective action and substantial effort.

143. What is the impact of the water crisis as mentioned in the first paragraph?
a. It promotes health and wellbeing.
b. It exacerbates poverty, creates health issues, and can trigger conflicts and migration.
c. It has no social implications.
d. It promotes international cooperation.

Answer: b. It exacerbates poverty, creates health issues, and can trigger conflicts and migration.

144. What does the passage imply about the role of technological innovation in addressing the water crisis?
a. It is the only solution to the crisis.
b. It is irrelevant.
c. It offers potential solutions, but it is not the only requirement.
d. It should be ignored.

Answer: c. It offers potential solutions, but it is not the only requirement.

145. Which of the following best summarizes the entire passage?
a. Water scarcity is an issue only faced by developing nations.
b. Technological innovation can solve the water crisis without any additional efforts.
c. The water crisis, impacting billions worldwide, requires sustainable management, technological innovation, and political action for resolution.
d. Water scarcity is primarily due to climate change.

Answer: c. The water crisis, impacting billions worldwide, requires sustainable management, technological innovation, and political action for resolution.

Passage: The global economy has witnessed a tremendous increase in the usage of cryptocurrencies. These digital assets, built on a technology called blockchain, promise a new era of decentralized financial transactions that could potentially render traditional banking systems obsolete. Bitcoin, the first and most popular cryptocurrency, has not only redefined the concept of money but has also sparked a whole new industry.

Cryptocurrencies operate independently of central banks and governments, offering a level of anonymity that has made them particularly appealing to certain sectors of society. The decentralized nature of these digital assets allows for a degree of freedom and flexibility not found in traditional financial systems.

However, cryptocurrencies also pose numerous challenges. Their value is notoriously volatile, and they have been associated with illicit activities due to their anonymous nature. Furthermore, while the technology underlying cryptocurrencies holds immense promise, it is still relatively new and unproven on a large scale.

Despite these challenges, the influence of cryptocurrencies on the global economy is growing. Some businesses are now accepting cryptocurrencies as payment, and various governments have begun exploring the potential of creating their own digital currencies. While it remains to be seen how cryptocurrencies will evolve, their impact on financial systems and society at large is undeniable.

146. What is the main topic of this passage?
a. The volatility of cryptocurrencies
b. The impact and influence of cryptocurrencies
c. The technology underlying cryptocurrencies
d. The association of cryptocurrencies with illicit activities

Answer: b. The impact and influence of cryptocurrencies

147. Which of the following best summarizes paragraph 2?
a. Cryptocurrencies are illegal.
b. Cryptocurrencies offer anonymity and operate independently of central banks, providing flexibility.
c. Cryptocurrencies are controlled by governments.
d. Cryptocurrencies are less flexible than traditional financial systems.

Answer: b. Cryptocurrencies offer anonymity and operate independently of central banks, providing flexibility.

148. What are the challenges associated with cryptocurrencies as mentioned in the passage?
a. They are not accepted by businesses.
b. Their value is volatile, and they can be associated with illicit activities.
c. They are controlled by central banks.
d. They are not built on blockchain technology.

Answer: b. Their value is volatile, and they can be associated with illicit activities.

149. Which detail is irrelevant to the main idea of paragraph 3?
a. Cryptocurrencies are notoriously volatile.
b. Cryptocurrencies have been associated with illicit activities.
c. The technology underlying cryptocurrencies is still relatively new.
d. Cryptocurrencies offer a level of anonymity.

Answer: d. Cryptocurrencies offer a level of anonymity.

150. What do some businesses and governments do in response to the influence of cryptocurrencies?
a. Some businesses accept cryptocurrencies as payment, and some governments explore creating their own digital currencies.
b. Businesses and governments reject cryptocurrencies.
c. Governments ban all cryptocurrencies.
d. Businesses stop accepting any form of digital payment.

Answer: a. Some businesses accept cryptocurrencies as payment, and some governments explore creating their own digital currencies.

151. Which of the following statements about Bitcoin is accurate according to the passage?
a. Bitcoin has redefined the concept of money and sparked a new industry.
b. Bitcoin is not a cryptocurrency.
c. Bitcoin is controlled by a central bank.
d. Bitcoin is less popular than other cryptocurrencies.

Answer: a. Bitcoin has redefined the concept of money and sparked a new industry.

152. What is the main idea of the final paragraph?
a. Cryptocurrencies have been banned globally.
b. Cryptocurrencies have no influence on the global economy.
c. Despite challenges, cryptocurrencies are growing in influence, with some businesses accepting them and governments exploring digital currencies.
d. The value of cryptocurrencies is very stable.

Answer: c. Despite challenges, cryptocurrencies are growing in influence, with some businesses accepting them and governments exploring digital currencies.

153. Which detail supports the idea that cryptocurrencies have a degree of freedom not found in traditional financial systems?
a. They are accepted by some businesses.
b. They are built on blockchain technology.
c. They operate independently of central banks.
d. They are associated with illicit activities.

Answer: c. They operate independently of central banks.

154. What does the passage imply about the future of cryptocurrencies?
a. They will be phased out soon.
b. They will replace all traditional banking systems.
c. They have the potential to evolve, but their exact future is uncertain.
d. They will become less popular over time.

Answer: c. They have the potential to evolve, but their exact future is uncertain.

155. Which of the following best summarizes the entire passage?
a. Cryptocurrencies are the future of all financial transactions.
b. Cryptocurrencies are causing major problems in the global economy.
c. The growth and influence of cryptocurrencies are undeniable, despite their challenges and the volatility associated with them.
d. Cryptocurrencies are only used for illicit activities.

Answer: c. The growth and influence of cryptocurrencies are undeniable, despite their challenges and the volatility associated with them.

Passage: As global temperatures rise, the Arctic ice has been melting at an alarming rate. This region, once a vast expanse of ice and snow, is rapidly transforming into a landscape of open water and tundra. The polar bear, one of the most iconic species of the Arctic, is now threatened by these changes.

These large, powerful creatures depend on sea ice for their survival. They hunt seals, their primary food source, from platforms of sea ice. As the ice melts, it becomes more difficult for polar bears to hunt and find food.

Consequently, many bears are forced to swim long distances in search of food and habitat. This often leads to exhaustion, and in some cases, death. Scientists are also noticing changes in polar bear behavior and biology as a response to their changing environment.

However, it's not all doom and gloom. Efforts to slow the melting of the Arctic ice are underway. Governments and environmental groups are working together to reduce greenhouse gas emissions, which are a major contributor to global warming. The outcome of these efforts is uncertain, but they offer a glimmer of hope for the future of the polar bear.

156. What is the primary focus of this passage?
a. The effect of global warming on polar bears
b. The effort to reduce greenhouse gas emissions
c. The transformation of the Arctic landscape
d. The biology and behavior of polar bears

Answer: a. The effect of global warming on polar bears

157. Which of the following best summarizes paragraph 2?
a. Polar bears have been forced to change their hunting habits due to the melting ice.
b. Polar bears are no longer able to find food.
c. Polar bears are moving to other habitats due to the melting ice.
d. Polar bears do not rely on sea ice for survival.

Answer: a. Polar bears have been forced to change their hunting habits due to the melting ice.

158. According to the passage, what is one consequence of the melting ice for polar bears?
a. They are growing larger.
b. They are forced to swim long distances, which can lead to exhaustion or death.
c. They are eating different types of food.
d. They are living longer.

Answer: b. They are forced to swim long distances, which can lead to exhaustion or death.

159. Which detail is irrelevant to the main idea of paragraph 3?
a. Polar bears are forced to swim long distances.
b. The long swims often lead to exhaustion and death.
c. Scientists are noticing changes in polar bear behavior and biology.
d. Efforts are underway to slow the melting of the Arctic ice.

Answer: d. Efforts are underway to slow the melting of the Arctic ice.

160. What are governments and environmental groups doing in response to the challenges faced by polar bears?
a. They are moving polar bears to new habitats.
b. They are working to reduce greenhouse gas emissions.
c. They are creating artificial platforms for polar bears to hunt from.
d. They are feeding the polar bears.

Answer: b. They are working to reduce greenhouse gas emissions.

161. What is the main food source of polar bears according to the passage?
a. Fish
b. Seals
c. Whales
d. Penguins

Answer: b. Seals

162. Which of the following best summarizes the last paragraph?
a. The polar bear population is rapidly increasing.
b. Efforts to reduce greenhouse gas emissions offer hope for the polar bears, despite the uncertain outcome.
c. The efforts to slow the Arctic ice melting have been successful.
d. Polar bears have adapted completely to the changing environment.

Answer: b. Efforts to reduce greenhouse gas emissions offer hope for the polar bears, despite the uncertain outcome.

Passage:

The internet has revolutionized modern communication. It has changed the way people work, study, shop, and interact. Social media platforms such as Facebook, Twitter, and Instagram have provided new avenues for expression and connection.

While the benefits are plentiful, the drawbacks of constant internet use are also becoming apparent. Research indicates that heavy internet use may lead to mental health issues like anxiety and depression, especially among teenagers. Moreover, privacy concerns due to data breaches have raised serious questions about the safety of sharing personal information online.

Artificial Intelligence is another emerging field impacted by the internet. AI algorithms learn from vast amounts of data collected online to make decisions and predictions, from recommending a movie on a streaming platform to assisting physicians in diagnosing diseases.

In summary, the internet, while revolutionary and beneficial in many ways, also brings about a unique set of challenges that society is still learning to navigate.

163. What is the main theme of this passage?
a. The impact of social media on teenagers
b. The use of Artificial Intelligence in healthcare
c. The benefits and challenges of the internet
d. Privacy concerns due to data breaches

Answer: c. The benefits and challenges of the internet

164. Which of the following best summarizes paragraph 2?
a. Data breaches have led to serious privacy concerns.
b. Heavy internet use can lead to mental health issues and privacy concerns.
c. The internet is leading to an increase in depression and anxiety among teenagers.
d. The use of social media platforms can lead to privacy breaches.

Answer: b. Heavy internet use can lead to mental health issues and privacy concerns.

165. According to the passage, how does AI learn to make decisions and predictions?
a. By studying human behavior
b. From vast amounts of data collected online
c. By interacting with other AI systems
d. By collecting personal information from social media

Answer: b. From vast amounts of data collected online

166. Which detail is irrelevant to the main idea of paragraph 3?
a. AI algorithms learn from online data.
b. AI assists physicians in diagnosing diseases.
c. Heavy internet use can lead to mental health issues.
d. AI can recommend movies on streaming platforms.

Answer: c. Heavy internet use can lead to mental health issues.

167. What are some of the ways the internet has changed modern life, according to the passage?
a. It has revolutionized communication, work, study, shopping, and social interaction.
b. It has led to a rise in mental health issues among teenagers.
c. It has made people more susceptible to data breaches.
d. It has decreased the privacy of personal information.

Answer: a. It has revolutionized communication, work, study, shopping, and social interaction.

168. Based on the passage, what is a potential downside of constant internet use?
a. It can lead to improved communication.
b. It can lead to mental health issues like anxiety and depression.
c. It can increase the efficiency of work and study.
d. It can provide new avenues for social connection.

Answer: b. It can lead to mental health issues like anxiety and depression.

169. Which of the following best summarizes the last paragraph?
a. The internet is revolutionary and beneficial in many ways but also brings about challenges.
b. The internet is only beneficial and has no challenges.
c. The challenges of the internet outweigh its benefits.
d. Society has successfully navigated the challenges brought about by the internet.

Answer: a. The internet is revolutionary and beneficial in many ways but also brings about challenges.

170. What is one application of AI mentioned in the passage?
a. Predicting weather patterns
b. Assisting physicians in diagnosing diseases
c. Driving autonomous vehicles
d. Cooking meals

Answer: b. Assisting physicians in diagnosing diseases

171. According to the passage, who is most at risk of developing mental health issues due to heavy internet use?
a. Elderly people
b. Teenagers
c. Physicians
d. AI researchers

Answer: b. Teenagers

172. Which social media platform is not mentioned in the passage?
a. Facebook
b. Twitter
c. LinkedIn
d. Instagram

Answer: c. LinkedIn

Passage: Evolving rapidly over the last decade, renewable energy sources such as solar, wind, and hydro power have become increasingly important in the global energy mix. The widespread adoption of renewable energy technologies has been driven by both environmental concerns and the economics of energy production.

Solar power, a form of renewable energy, harnesses sunlight to generate electricity. Photovoltaic cells convert sunlight directly into electricity, while concentrated solar power systems use mirrors or lenses to focus sunlight onto a small area, generating heat that is used to produce electricity.

Wind power, another form of renewable energy, utilizes the kinetic energy of wind to generate electricity. Wind turbines, which convert wind energy into mechanical energy, are used in both onshore and offshore settings.

Hydro power, which has been used for centuries, involves harnessing the energy of moving water to generate electricity. Traditional hydroelectric power plants use a dam on a river to store water, which is released to turn a turbine, generating electricity.

The transition towards renewable energy sources presents both challenges and opportunities. While these sources reduce our reliance on fossil fuels and decrease greenhouse gas emissions, they also require significant infrastructure investments and pose issues such as intermittent supply.

173. What is the main idea of the passage?
a. The workings of solar power
b. The evolution and significance of renewable energy sources
c. The economics of energy production
d. The environmental concerns related to renewable energy sources

Answer: b. The evolution and significance of renewable energy sources

174. Which of the following best summarizes the second paragraph?
a. Solar power utilizes mirrors and lenses to focus sunlight.
b. Solar power uses photovoltaic cells and concentrated solar power systems to generate electricity.
c. Solar power has become the most important source of renewable energy.
d. Solar power harnesses sunlight to generate electricity using different systems.

Answer: d. Solar power harnesses sunlight to generate electricity using different systems.

175. How does wind power generate electricity, according to the passage?
a. By harnessing the kinetic energy of wind
b. By using mirrors or lenses to focus wind energy
c. By using a dam on a river to store wind
d. By converting sunlight directly into electricity

Answer: a. By harnessing the kinetic energy of wind

176. Which detail is irrelevant to the main idea of the third paragraph?
a. Wind power utilizes the kinetic energy of wind.
b. Wind turbines convert wind energy into mechanical energy.
c. Wind turbines are used in both onshore and offshore settings.
d. Wind power uses a dam on a river to store wind.

Answer: d. Wind power uses a dam on a river to store wind.

177. What is one challenge of transitioning towards renewable energy sources mentioned in the passage?
a. It increases reliance on fossil fuels.
b. It requires significant infrastructure investments.
c. It eliminates all environmental concerns.
d. It decreases greenhouse gas emissions.

Answer: b. It requires significant infrastructure investments.

178. How does hydro power generate electricity, according to the passage?
a. By harnessing the energy of moving water
b. By focusing sunlight onto a small area
c. By using the kinetic energy of wind
d. By converting sunlight directly into electricity

Answer: a. By harnessing the energy of moving water

179. Which of the following best summarizes the last paragraph?
a. The transition towards renewable energy sources is free from challenges.
b. Renewable energy sources decrease greenhouse gas emissions but require infrastructure investments.
c. Renewable energy sources only pose issues of intermittent supply.
d. Renewable energy sources are economically not viable.

Answer: b. Renewable energy sources decrease greenhouse gas emissions but require infrastructure investments.

180. What is not a form of renewable energy mentioned in the passage?
a. Solar power
b. Wind power
c. Nuclear power
d. Hydro power

Answer: c. Nuclear power

181. How does a traditional hydroelectric power plant generate electricity, according to the passage?
a. By using a dam on a river to store water which is released to turn a turbine
b. By harnessing the kinetic energy of wind
c. By using photovoltaic cells to convert sunlight directly into electricity
d. By using mirrors or lenses to focus sunlight onto a small area

Answer: a. By using a dam on a river to store water which is released to turn a turbine

182. What has driven the adoption of renewable energy technologies, according to the passage?
a. Only environmental concerns
b. Only economics of energy production
c. Both environmental concerns and the economics of energy production
d. Neither environmental concerns nor the economics of energy production

Answer: c. Both environmental concerns and the economics of energy production

Passage: The ancient city of Rome, founded in 753 BC according to tradition, was originally a small agricultural community on the banks of the Tiber River. Over the centuries, it grew into a vast empire, covering much of Europe, North Africa, and the Middle East.

The Roman Empire was known for its exceptional administrative system, advanced engineering, and contributions to arts and culture. The Romans built impressive structures like aqueducts, amphitheaters, and roads that are still in use today. The Roman language, Latin, influenced many modern languages and Roman law forms the basis of legal systems in many western countries.

The fall of the Roman Empire in 476 AD, marked by the deposition of the last Roman emperor, Romulus Augustus, was due to a combination of internal strife, economic instability, and pressure from barbarian invasions. Despite its downfall, Rome's influence on western civilization is profound and lasting.

The city today, known as the 'Eternal City', is a vibrant mix of ruins, art, history, street life, and culture – an embodiment of the Roman 'dolce vita' or 'sweet life'. Tourists are drawn to the remnants of the city's imperial glory, like the Colosseum, the Roman Forum, and the Pantheon.

183. What is the main idea of the passage?
a. The growth and influence of ancient Rome
b. The fall of the Roman Empire
c. The modern city of Rome
d. The Roman contributions to arts and culture

Answer: a. The growth and influence of ancient Rome

184. Which of the following best summarizes the first paragraph?
a. Rome was a small agricultural community that transformed into a vast empire.
b. Rome was founded on the banks of the Tiber River.
c. Rome covered much of Europe, North Africa, and the Middle East.
d. Rome was an ancient city founded in 753 BC.

Answer: a. Rome was a small agricultural community that transformed into a vast empire.

185. Which of the following was not mentioned as a contribution of the Roman Empire?
a. Advanced engineering
b. An exceptional administrative system
c. The development of the Latin language
d. Invention of the printing press

Answer: d. Invention of the printing press

186. Which detail is irrelevant to the main idea of the fourth paragraph?
a. The city today is known as the 'Eternal City'.
b. Tourists are drawn to the remnants of the city's imperial glory.
c. The last Roman emperor was Romulus Augustus.
d. The city is an embodiment of the Roman 'dolce vita' or 'sweet life'.

Answer: c. The last Roman emperor was Romulus Augustus.

187. According to the passage, what was a reason for the fall of the Roman Empire?
a. Lack of impressive structures
b. Pressure from barbarian invasions
c. Loss of agricultural land
d. Decline in the use of the Latin language

Answer: b. Pressure from barbarian invasions

188. What was a significant influence of the Romans on modern languages?
a. The Romans invented many modern languages.
b. The Romans influenced many modern languages through Latin.
c. The Roman language was adopted by many modern countries.
d. The Romans created a universal language.

Answer: b. The Romans influenced many modern languages through Latin.

189. Which of the following best summarizes the third paragraph?
a. The Romans built aqueducts, amphitheaters, and roads.
b. The Roman Empire was known for its administrative system, advanced engineering, and cultural contributions.
c. Roman law forms the basis of legal systems in many western countries.
d. The Roman language, Latin, was the most spoken language in the world.

Answer: b. The Roman Empire was known for its administrative system, advanced engineering, and cultural contributions.

190. How is Rome described in the present day?
a. A small agricultural community
b. A city suffering from economic instability
c. A city of ruins, art, history, and vibrant street life
d. A city under pressure from barbarian invasions

Answer: c. A city of ruins, art, history, and vibrant street life

191. Which of the following structures is not listed in the passage as a Roman architectural marvel?
a. Colosseum
b. Roman Forum
c. Eiffel Tower
d. Pantheon

Answer: c. Eiffel Tower

192. What phrase is used to embody the life in modern Rome?
a. 'Eternal City'
b. 'Dolce vita'
c. 'Imperial glory'
d. 'Fall of the Roman Empire'

Answer: b. 'Dolce vita'

Passage:Jane was tired of the rat race, of the nine-to-five grind. She had worked in the city for more than twenty years and she was done. She had a dream of a quieter, more peaceful life. A life on the coast where she could breathe the salty air and listen to the waves lapping against the shore. The decision wasn't easy, but she was resolute. She would give it all up, buy a little house by the sea, and live the life she had always wanted.

193. Which of the following best represents the tone of this passage?
a. Anxious and regretful
b. Confident and hopeful
c. Resentful and angry
d. Disappointed and resigned

Answer: b. Confident and hopeful
Explanation: The language and descriptions in this passage suggest a tone of confidence and hope. Jane is tired of her current life but she is decisive ("resolute") about pursuing her dream. She envisions a more peaceful life and is ready to make a change to achieve it.

194. Given the information in the passage, which conclusion could you draw about Jane?
a. She dislikes her current job.
b. She lives near the sea.
c. She has always lived in the city.
d. She has family living on the coast.

Answer: a. She dislikes her current job.
Explanation: The passage indicates that Jane is "tired of the rat race" and "done" with working in the city, which implies a dislike for her current job. The other options are not explicitly or implicitly supported by the passage.

195. What can be inferred about Jane's emotional state from the passage?
a. She is scared about the future.
b. She is excited about her decision.
c. She is indifferent to her current situation.
d. She is confused about what to do next.

Answer: b. She is excited about her decision.
Explanation: Although the passage does not explicitly state Jane's emotional state, the tone and content suggest that she feels hopeful and confident about her decision to move to the coast.

196. What does the phrase "rat race" in the passage most likely refer to?
a. A literal competition involving rats
b. The competitive nature of city life
c. A hobby Jane used to enjoy
d. Jane's daily commute to work

Answer: b. The competitive nature of city life
Explanation: The term "rat race" is commonly used to describe the relentless, competitive struggle for success in work or business, typically in a city or high-stress environment.

197. Which statement would the author most likely agree with based on the passage?
a. Everyone should quit their jobs and move to the coast.
b. Living in the city is a terrible experience.
c. It is important to pursue your dreams.
d. Jane is making a rash decision.

Answer: c. It is important to pursue your dreams.
Explanation: The author describes Jane's decision to pursue her dream of living by the sea in a positive light, suggesting an endorsement of the idea that pursuing personal dreams is important. The other options make broader or more negative claims that are not supported by the passage.

Passage: Dr. Morrison was a quintessential academic. Always found buried in stacks of books, she had an insatiable thirst for knowledge. She was a polymath, her interests spanning from astronomy to zoology. Her colleagues often called her a "walking encyclopedia", as she was always ready to share a fascinating tidbit or clarify a complex concept.

198. In the context of the passage, what does "quintessential" likely mean?
a. Controversial
b. Representative
c. Eccentric
d. Overbearing

Answer: b. Representative
Explanation: The word "quintessential" is used to describe something or someone that is a perfect example or embodiment of a quality or type. In this context, Dr. Morrison is described as the perfect example of an academic, as shown by her thirst for knowledge and wide-ranging interests.

199. In the passage, the term "polymath" most likely means a person who is:
a. Fluent in many languages
b. Skilled in physical activities
c. Interested in many areas of knowledge
d. Able to do complex mathematical calculations

Answer: c. Interested in many areas of knowledge
Explanation: A "polymath" is a person of wide knowledge or learning. The context makes clear that Dr. Morrison's interests span a range of subjects, which supports this definition.

200. What does the phrase "walking encyclopedia" suggest about Dr. Morrison?
a. She is very old.
b. She has a photographic memory.
c. She has a broad range of knowledge.
d. She is a published author.

Answer: c. She has a broad range of knowledge
Explanation: A "walking encyclopedia" is a person who has a large amount of knowledge. The phrase is used here to emphasize Dr. Morrison's extensive knowledge across different fields.

201. In the context of the passage, the word "insatiable" most likely means:
a. Irritating
b. Impossible to satisfy
c. Incomplete
d. Non-stop

Answer: b. Impossible to satisfy
Explanation: In this context, "insatiable" describes Dr. Morrison's thirst for knowledge, implying that it cannot be fully satisfied - she always wants to learn more.

202. Based on the passage, what does "tidbit" likely mean?
a. A small piece of interesting information
b. A small snack
c. A difficult problem
d. A rare book

Answer: a. A small piece of interesting information
Explanation: In this context, "tidbit" is used to describe the interesting pieces of information that Dr. Morrison is always ready to share. This suggests that it refers to a small piece of interesting information rather than the other options.

203. Which of the following is equal to the rational number -3/4?
a. 0.75
b. -0.75
c. -1.75
d. 1.75

Answer: b. -0.75
Explanation: The rational number -3/4 is equal to -0.75 when converted to decimal form.

204. If you subtract the rational number -1/2 from 1/4, what is the result?
a. -1/4
b. 1/2
c. 3/4
d. -3/4

Answer: c. 3/4
Explanation: When you subtract -1/2, it's the same as adding 1/2. Therefore, 1/4 + 1/2 equals 3/4.

205. What is the product of the rational numbers -3/5 and 2/3?
a. 1
b. -1
c. -6/15
d. 6/15

Answer: c. -6/15
Explanation: The product of -3/5 and 2/3 is -6/15, which can be simplified to -2/5.

206. Which of the following rational numbers is the largest?
a. -3/4
b. -5/6
c. -2/3
d. -7/8

Answer: c. -2/3
Explanation: When comparing negative fractions, the fraction closest to zero is the largest. So, -2/3 is the largest among the options.

207. If you divide the rational number 5/6 by 2/3, what is the result?
a. 1 1/4
b. 1 1/2
c. 1 3/4
d. 2

Answer: d. 2
Explanation: Dividing by a fraction is the same as multiplying by its reciprocal. The reciprocal of 2/3 is 3/2, and 5/6 multiplied by 3/2 equals 2.

208. What is the result when the rational number 2/3 is raised to the power of 2?
a. 1/3
b. 2/3
c. 4/9
d. 1 1/3

Answer: c. 4/9. Explanation: When you raise 2/3 to the power of 2, you square both the numerator and the denominator, resulting in 4/9.

209. What is the result when the rational number 1/2 is subtracted from 2/3?
a. 1/2
b. 1/3
c. 1/6
d. 2/3

Answer: c. 1/6
Explanation: When you subtract 1/2 from 2/3, you get 1/6.

210. What is the result of adding the rational numbers -2/3 and -1/2?
a. -1 1/6
b. -1/6
c. 1/6
d. 1 1/6

Answer: a. -1 1/6
Explanation: The sum of -2/3 and -1/2 is -1 1/6.

211. Which of the following rational numbers is equal to 75%?
a. 3/4
b. 7/8
c. 5/6
d. 2/3

Answer: a. 3/4
Explanation: 75% as a fraction is 3/4.

212. What is the result when the rational number -2/3 is multiplied by -3/4?
a. 1/2
b. 1
c. 1 1/2
d. 2

Answer: b. 1
Explanation: The product of -2/3 and -3/4 is 1, as the negatives cancel each other out.

213. Which of the following is a rational number?
a. $\sqrt{2}$
b. π
c. 3/2
d. $\sqrt{-1}$

Answer: c. 3/2
Explanation: A rational number can be expressed as a fraction where both the numerator and the denominator are integers. The numbers $\sqrt{2}$ and π are irrational because they cannot be expressed as a simple fraction, and $\sqrt{-1}$ is an imaginary number.

214. How does a rational number differ from an integer?
a. Rational numbers can be negative, but integers can't.
b. Rational numbers can be fractions, but integers can't.
c. Rational numbers can't be fractions, but integers can.
d. There is no difference; all integers are rational numbers.

Answer: b. Rational numbers can be fractions, but integers can't.
Explanation: While all integers are also considered rational numbers, not all rational numbers are integers because rational numbers can be fractions.

215. A nurse needs to administer 1.5 liters of saline solution to a patient over 4 hours. How many liters per hour should the nurse administer?
a. 0.25 liters
b. 0.375 liters
c. 0.5 liters
d. 0.75 liters

Answer: c. 0.5 liters
Explanation: To find the hourly rate, divide the total volume by the total time. 1.5 liters divided by 4 hours equals 0.5 liters per hour.

216. In a clinical lab, the normal range of a particular blood parameter is 0.7 to 1.2. This range represents:
a. Integers
b. Whole numbers
c. Irrational numbers
d. Rational numbers

Answer: d. Rational numbers
Explanation: The range 0.7 to 1.2 represents rational numbers as these numbers can be expressed as fractions (7/10 to 6/5).

217. The decimal number 0.75 can also be expressed as:
a. 75%
b. 7.5%
c. 750%
d. 75/1000

Answer: a. 75%
Explanation: The decimal 0.75 is equivalent to 75/100 or 75%.

218. If a physician orders 0.5 grams of a medication and the medication is available in 250 milligram tablets, how many tablets should be administered?
a. 1 tablet
b. 2 tablets
c. 3 tablets
d. 4 tablets

Answer: b. 2 tablets
Explanation: 0.5 grams is equal to 500 milligrams. Therefore, 500 milligrams divided by 250 milligrams per tablet equals 2 tablets.

219. The number 5.678 is a(n):
a. Integer
b. Irrational number
c. Rational number
d. Imaginary number

Answer: c. Rational number
Explanation: This number can be expressed as a simple fraction (5678/1000), so it is a rational number.

220. In a prescription, a medication is to be given in a dosage of 3/4 mg. This dosage represents a:
a. Whole number
b. Integer
c. Rational number
d. Irrational number

Answer: c. Rational number. Explanation: 3/4 is a rational number as it can be expressed as a fraction where the numerator and the denominator are integers.

221. The ratio of nurses to patients in a clinic is 5 to 100. This ratio represents a:
a. Whole number
b. Integer
c. Rational number
d. Irrational number

Answer: c. Rational number. Explanation: The ratio 5 to 100 can be expressed as the fraction 5/100, which is a rational number.

222. The square root of which of the following numbers is a rational number?
a. 2
b. 3
c. 4
d. 5

Answer: c. 4

Explanation: The square root of 4 is 2, which is a rational number because it can be expressed as the fraction 2/1.

223. If 2x + 3 = 11, what is the value of x?
a. 2
b. 3
c. 4
d. 5

Answer: c. 4

Explanation: Subtract 3 from both sides of the equation to get 2x = 8. Then, divide both sides by 2 to find that x = 4.

224. Consider the equation 4x - 2 = 14. What is the value of x?
a. 3
b. 4
c. 5
d. 6

Answer: b. 4

Explanation: Add 2 to both sides of the equation to get 4x = 16. Then, divide both sides by 4 to find that x = 4.

225. In the equation 3x + 4 = 10, what is the value of x?
a. 1
b. 2
c. 3
d. 4

Answer: b. 2

Explanation: Subtract 4 from both sides of the equation to get 3x = 6. Then, divide both sides by 3 to find that x = 2.

226. The equation 5x - 7 = 8 can be solved to find the value of x. What is it?
a. 1
b. 2
c. 3
d. 4

Answer: c. 3

Explanation: Add 7 to both sides of the equation to get 5x = 15. Then, divide both sides by 5 to find that x = 3.

227. For the equation 4x + 2 = 3x + 5, what is the value of x?
a. 1
b. 2
c. 3
d. 4

Answer: c. 3
Explanation: Subtract 3x from both sides to get x + 2 = 5. Then subtract 2 from both sides to find x = 3.

228. In the equation 3(x - 2) = 9, what is the value of x?
a. 3
b. 4
c. 5
d. 6

Answer: c. 5
Explanation: Divide both sides by 3 to get x - 2 = 3. Then, add 2 to both sides to find that x = 5.

229. Consider the equation 2(x + 3) = 10. What is the value of x?
a. 1
b. 2
c. 3
d. 4

Answer: b. 2
Explanation: Divide both sides by 2 to get x + 3 = 5. Then, subtract 3 from both sides to find that x = 2.

230. For the equation 5(x - 2) + 3 = 18, what is the value of x?
a. 3
b. 4
c. 5
d. 6

Answer: b. 4
Explanation: Subtract 3 from both sides to get 5(x - 2) = 15. Then divide by 5 to get x - 2 = 3, and finally add 2 to both sides to find x = 4.

231. In the equation 2x - 3 = 3(x - 2), what is the value of x?
a. 1
b. 3
c. 5
d. 7

Answer: b. 3
Explanation: Simplify the right side of the equation to get 2x - 3 = 3x - 6. Then subtract 2x from both sides to get -3 = x - 6. Finally, add 6 to both sides to find x = 3.

232. For the equation x/2 + 3 = 6, what is the value of x?
a. 2
b. 4
c. 6
d. 8

Answer: d. 8
Explanation: Subtract 3 from both sides to get x/2 = 3. Then, multiply both sides by 2 to find that x = 8.

233. A patient needs to be given 8mg of a medication per kilogram of body weight. The patient weighs 75kg. How much medication should they receive?
a. 400mg
b. 500mg
c. 600mg
d. 700mg

Answer: c. 600mg
Explanation: Use the equation (8mg/kg)(75kg) = 600mg.

234. The recommended dosage of a medication is 10mg/kg body weight. If a patient weighs 50kg, how much medication should be administered?
a. 400mg
b. 500mg
c. 600mg
d. 700mg

Answer: b. 500mg
Explanation: Using the equation (10mg/kg)(50kg) = 500mg.

235. A patient's blood sugar level needs to be maintained at around 120mg/dL. If their current level is 170mg/dL, what is the percentage decrease required?
a. 22%
b. 27%
c. 29%
d. 35%

Answer: c. 29%
Explanation: The decrease required is 170mg/dL - 120mg/dL = 50mg/dL. As a percentage of the initial level, this is (50/170)*100 = 29.41%, approximately 29%.

244. If p is a prime number and q is an integer, which of the following must be a rational number?
a. p/q
b. p^q
c. q^p
d. √p

Answer: a. p/q
Explanation: A rational number is defined as a number that can be expressed in the form p/q, where p and q are integers and q ≠ 0. Thus, p/q is a rational number.

245. Which of the following expressions must be a rational number?
a. The sum of two irrational numbers
b. The product of two irrational numbers
c. The difference between two irrational numbers
d. All of the above

Answer: d. All of the above
Explanation: The sum, product, or difference of two irrational numbers can be a rational number.

246. Which of the following is an example of a rational number?
a. The square root of 2
b. The square root of -1
c. The ratio of the circumference of a circle to its diameter
d. The number -7/3

Answer: d. The number -7/3
Explanation: A rational number is a number that can be expressed as a fraction p/q, where p and q are integers and q ≠ 0. Therefore, -7/3 is a rational number.

247. Which of the following is a rational number?
a. The number π (Pi)
b. The square root of 3
c. The number 0
d. The natural logarithm of 2 (ln 2)

Answer: c. The number 0. Explanation: Zero is a rational number because it can be expressed as 0/1, which fits the definition of a rational number.

248. Which of the following statements is true about rational numbers?
a. All rational numbers are integers
b. All integers are rational numbers
c. All real numbers are rational numbers
d. All irrational numbers are rational numbers

Answer: b. All integers are rational numbers
Explanation: All integers can be expressed as a fraction with 1 in the denominator, which makes them rational numbers.

249. If x and y are integers and y ≠ 0, which of the following must be a rational number?
a. x^y
b. y^x
c. x/y
d. x + y

Answer: c. x/y
Explanation: A rational number is a number that can be expressed in the form p/q, where p and q are integers and q ≠ 0. Thus, x/y is a rational number.

250. Which of the following numbers is not a rational number?
a. 1/3
b. 0.5
c. √4
d. √3

Answer: d. √3
Explanation: The square root of 3 cannot be written as a fraction of two integers, making it an irrational number.

251. Which of the following expressions must be a rational number?
a. The sum of two rational numbers
b. The product of two rational numbers
c. The difference between two rational numbers
d. All of the above

Answer: d. All of the above
Explanation: The sum, product, or difference of two rational numbers is always a rational number.

252. Which of the following numbers is a rational number?
a. √2
b. π (Pi)
c. e (Euler's Number)
d. -5/2

Answer: d. -5/2
Explanation: A rational number can be expressed as a fraction of two integers. -5/2 fits this definition, so it is a rational number.

252. Given the rational numbers 3/4 and 1/2, what is their sum?
a. 5/8
b. 1/4
c. 1 1/4
d. 1

Answer: c. 1 1/4
Explanation: To add fractions, you need a common denominator. In this case, the common denominator is 4. So, 3/4 + 2/4 (which is 1/2 in terms of fourths) equals 5/4 or 1 1/4.

253. What is the product of the rational numbers -5/6 and 4/3?
a. -10/3
b. -10/9
c. -20/18
d. -20/9

Answer: a. -10/3
Explanation: When you multiply fractions, you simply multiply the numerators together and the denominators together. -5/6 * 4/3 = -20/18 which simplifies to -10/9.

254. What is the result of subtracting the rational number 2/3 from 5/6?
a. 1/6
b. 1/3
c. 1/2
d. 2/3

Answer: a. 1/6. Explanation: To subtract fractions, you need a common denominator. In this case, the common denominator is 6. So, 5/6 - 4/6 (which is 2/3 in terms of sixths) equals 1/6.

255. Given the rational numbers 3/4 and 1/2, what is their quotient?
a. 1/2
b. 2/3
c. 3/2
d. 3/8

Answer: c. 3/2. Explanation: When you divide fractions, you multiply the first fraction by the reciprocal of the second. So, 3/4 ÷ 1/2 = 3/4 * 2/1 = 3/2.

256. What is the result of adding the rational numbers -3/5 and 1/4?
a. -17/20
b. 1/9
c. 7/20
d. -7/20

Answer: d. -7/20

Explanation: To add fractions, you need a common denominator. In this case, the common denominator is 20. So, -12/20 (which is -3/5 in terms of twentieths) + 5/20 (which is 1/4 in terms of twentieths) equals -7/20.

257. What is the product of the rational numbers 2/3 and -3/4?
a. 1/2
b. -1/2
c. -3/2
d. -1/3

Answer: b. -1/2

Explanation: When you multiply fractions, you simply multiply the numerators together and the denominators together. 2/3 * -3/4 = -6/12 which simplifies to -1/2.

258. What is the result of subtracting the rational number -1/2 from -2/3?
a. -1/6
b. 1/6
c. -1/3
d. 1/3

Answer: a. -1/6

Explanation: To subtract fractions, you need a common denominator. In this case, the common denominator is 6. So, -4/6 (which is -2/3 in terms of sixths) - -3/6 (which is -1/2 in terms of sixths) equals -1/6.

259. What is the quotient of the rational numbers -6/7 and 2/3?
a. 9/7
b. -9/7
c. -9/14
d. -18/14

Answer: b. -9/7

Explanation: When you divide fractions, you multiply the first fraction by the reciprocal of the second. So, -6/7 ÷ 2/3 = -6/7 * 3/2 = -18/14, which simplifies to -9/7.

260. What is the result of adding the rational numbers 4/5 and -3/10?
a. 1/10
b. 1/2
c. 2/5
d. -2/5

Answer: c. 2/5
Explanation: To add fractions, you need a common denominator. In this case, the common denominator is 10. So, 8/10 (which is 4/5 in terms of tenths) + -3/10 equals 5/10, which simplifies to 1/2.

261. What is the product of the rational numbers -5/8 and -2/3?
a. 5/12
b. -5/12
c. 10/24
d. -10/24

Answer: a. 5/12
Explanation: When you multiply fractions, you simply multiply the numerators together and the denominators together. -5/8 * -2/3 = 10/24 which simplifies to 5/12.

262. When solving the equation 2x - 3 = 11, which is the first step?
a. Add 3 to both sides.
b. Divide both sides by 2.
c. Subtract 11 from both sides.
d. Multiply both sides by 2.

Answer: a. Add 3 to both sides.
Explanation: The first step in solving this equation would be to isolate the term with the variable. You can do this by adding 3 to both sides of the equation, which results in 2x = 14.

263. The equation 5(x - 2) = 15 is given. What is the first step to solve it?
a. Multiply the 5 into the parentheses.
b. Divide both sides by 5.
c. Subtract 2 from both sides.
d. Add 2 to both sides.

Answer: a. Multiply the 5 into the parentheses.
Explanation: The first step in solving this equation is to distribute the 5 into the parentheses, resulting in 5x - 10 = 15.

264. Given the equation 3x + 5 = 2x + 10, what should be the first step to solve it?
a. Subtract 2x from both sides.
b. Subtract 3x from both sides.
c. Subtract 5 from both sides.
d. Add 5 to both sides.

Answer: a. Subtract 2x from both sides.
Explanation: The first step to solve this equation would be to get all the x terms on one side. This can be achieved by subtracting 2x from both sides, resulting in x + 5 = 10.

265. When solving the equation 4x = 16, what should you do first?
a. Add 16 to both sides.
b. Subtract 4 from both sides.
c. Divide both sides by 4.
d. Multiply both sides by 4.

Answer: c. Divide both sides by 4.
Explanation: To solve for x, you need to isolate it. Divide both sides by 4, which will give you x = 4.

266. Given the equation 2(x - 3) + 5 = 13, which step should you do first?
a. Distribute the 2 into the parentheses.
b. Subtract 5 from both sides.
c. Divide both sides by 2.
d. Add 3 to both sides.

Answer: a. Distribute the 2 into the parentheses.
Explanation: The first step to solve this equation is to distribute the 2 into the parentheses, which results in 2x - 6 + 5 = 13.

267. When given the equation 3(2x - 1) = 18, what is the first step to solve it?
a. Divide both sides by 3.
b. Multiply the 3 into the parentheses.
c. Add 1 to both sides.
d. Subtract 18 from both sides.

Answer: b. Multiply the 3 into the parentheses.
Explanation: The first step to solve this equation is to distribute the 3 into the parentheses, which gives 6x - 3 = 18.

268. Given the equation x/4 + 2 = 5, which step should you do first?
a. Subtract 2 from both sides.
b. Add 2 to both sides.
c. Multiply both sides by 4.
d. Divide both sides by 4.

Answer: a. Subtract 2 from both sides. Explanation: The first step in solving this equation would be to isolate the term with the variable. This can be done by subtracting 2 from both sides, giving x/4 = 3.

269. For the equation 5x - 2 = 3x + 4, what should be the first step to solve it?
a. Subtract 3x from both sides.
b. Subtract 5x from both sides.
c. Add 2 to both sides.
d. Subtract 2 from both sides.

Answer: a. Subtract 3x from both sides.
Explanation: The first step to solve this equation would be to get all the x terms on one side. This can be achieved by subtracting 3x from both sides, resulting in 2x - 2 = 4.

270. When given the equation 7 = 2x + 1, what is the first step to solve it?
a. Subtract 1 from both sides.
b. Subtract 7 from both sides.
c. Divide both sides by 2.
d. Add 1 to both sides.

Answer: a. Subtract 1 from both sides.
Explanation: The first step to solve this equation would be to isolate the term with the variable. You can do this by subtracting 1 from both sides, which results in 6 = 2x.

271. For the equation 4(x + 2) - 3 = 17, what should you do first?
a. Add 3 to both sides.
b. Subtract 4 from both sides.
c. Distribute the 4 into the parentheses.
d. Divide both sides by 4.

Answer: c. Distribute the 4 into the parentheses.
Explanation: The first step to solve this equation is to distribute the 4 into the parentheses, resulting in 4x + 8 - 3 = 17.

272. A nurse is calculating the dosage of a medication for a patient. The standard dosage is 5 mg/kg. The patient weighs 75 kg. The equation 5x = 375 represents this situation. What does x represent in this equation?
a. The weight of the patient.
b. The standard dosage.
c. The total dosage for the patient.
d. The weight of the medication.

Answer: c. The total dosage for the patient.
Explanation: In this equation, x represents the total dosage of the medication for the patient. By solving the equation, we find that x equals 75, which means the patient should receive a total of 75 mg of the medication.

273. Given the equation 2(x + 3) = 20, what is the solution for x?
a. 5
b. 7
c. 10
d. 14

Answer: b. 7
Explanation: First, distribute the 2 in the parentheses to get 2x + 6 = 20. Then subtract 6 from both sides to get 2x = 14. Finally, divide both sides by 2 to solve for x, which gives x = 7.

274. Given the equation 4x - 2 = 2x + 8, what is the solution for x?
a. 2
b. 5
c. 7
d. 10

Answer: b. 5
Explanation: First, subtract 2x from both sides to get 2x - 2 = 8. Then add 2 to both sides to get 2x = 10. Finally, divide both sides by 2 to solve for x, which gives x = 5.

275. Given the equation 3(x - 2) + 4 = 10, what is the solution for x?
a. 1
b. 2
c. 3
d. 4

Answer: c. 3
Explanation: First, distribute the 3 in the parentheses to get 3x - 6 + 4 = 10. Simplify to get 3x - 2 = 10. Then add 2 to both sides to get 3x = 12. Finally, divide both sides by 3 to solve for x, which gives x = 4.

276. Consider the equation 5(x - 1) = 3(x + 2). What is the solution for x?
a. 2
b. 3
c. 4
d. 5

Answer: a. 2
Explanation: First, distribute on both sides to get 5x - 5 = 3x + 6. Subtract 3x from both sides to get 2x - 5 = 6. Add 5 to both sides to get 2x = 11. Finally, divide by 2 on both sides to get x = 5.5.

277. Given the equation x/3 + 2 = 4, what is the solution for x?
a. 2
b. 4
c. 6
d. 9

Answer: c. 6
Explanation: First, subtract 2 from both sides to get x/3 = 2. Multiply by 3 on both sides to solve for x, which gives x = 6.

278. Consider the equation x/2 - 3 = 2. What is the solution for x?
a. 4
b. 6
c. 8
d. 10

Answer: d. 10
Explanation: First, add 3 to both sides to get x/2 = 5. Multiply by 2 on both sides to solve for x, which gives x = 10.

279. Given the quadratic equation x^2 - 5x + 6 = 0, what are the solutions for x?
a. x = 1 and x = 4
b. x = 2 and x = 3
c. x = -2 and x = -3
d. x = 1 and x = 6

Answer: b. x = 2 and x = 3
Explanation: This quadratic equation can be factored to (x - 2)(x - 3) = 0. Setting each factor equal to zero gives the solutions x = 2 and x = 3.

280. Given the quadratic equation x^2 + 5x + 6 = 0, what are the solutions for x?
a. x = -2 and x = -3
b. x = 2 and x = 3
c. x = -1 and x = -6
d. x = 1 and x = 6

Answer: a. x = -2 and x = -3
Explanation: This quadratic equation can be factored to (x + 2)(x + 3) = 0. Setting each factor equal to zero gives the solutions x = -2 and x = -3.

281. Given the equation x^2 = 25, what are the solutions for x?
a. x = 5
b. x = -5
c. x = 5 and x = -5
d. There are no solutions.

Answer: c. x = 5 and x = -5
Explanation: When you take the square root of both sides of the equation, you get x = 5 and x = -5. The square root of a number has two values, positive and negative, so there are two solutions for x in this equation.

282. A nurse needs to administer a medication that has a recommended dosage of 2 mg per 10 kg of body weight. If a patient weighs 60 kg, how much of the medication should the patient receive?
a. 6 mg
b. 12 mg
c. 15 mg
d. 20 mg

Answer: b. 12 mg
Explanation: The ratio of medication to body weight is 2:10. If the patient weighs 60 kg, then the medication dosage is 2*(60/10) = 12 mg.

283. A pediatric nurse notices that 4 out of 5 children prefer flavored medicine to unflavored. What percentage of children prefer flavored medicine?
a. 50%
b. 60%
c. 80%
d. 100%

Answer: c. 80%
Explanation: The ratio of children who prefer flavored medicine to the total is 4:5. This ratio translates to 80%.

284. A nurse is reading a patient's lab results. The patient's LDL cholesterol to HDL cholesterol ratio is 3:1. What does this mean?
a. The patient's LDL cholesterol is three times higher than their HDL cholesterol.
b. The patient's HDL cholesterol is three times higher than their LDL cholesterol.
c. The patient's total cholesterol is 3.
d. The patient's total cholesterol is 1.

Answer: a. The patient's LDL cholesterol is three times higher than their HDL cholesterol.
Explanation: A 3:1 ratio means that for every three parts of one thing, there is one part of another. In this case, the patient's LDL cholesterol is three times higher than their HDL cholesterol.

285. A nurse calculates that a patient's intake of fluids is 2500 mL and their output is 2200 mL over 24 hours. What is the net fluid balance?
a. 200 mL
b. 300 mL
c. 400 mL
d. 500 mL

Answer: b. 300 mL
Explanation: The net fluid balance is calculated by subtracting the fluid output from the fluid input. In this case, 2500 mL - 2200 mL = 300 mL.

286. A nurse is reviewing lab results and notes that a patient's sodium to potassium ratio is 20:1. This ratio is unusually high, as a healthy ratio is closer to 14:1. What percentage higher is the patient's ratio compared to a healthy ratio?
a. 20%
b. 30%
c. 42.86%
d. 50%

Answer: c. 42.86%
Explanation: The percentage difference between the patient's ratio and a healthy ratio is calculated as (20-14)/14 * 100 = 42.86%.

287. In a nursing home with 100 residents, 25 residents have been diagnosed with diabetes. What is the percentage of nursing home residents diagnosed with diabetes?
a. 10%
b. 15%
c. 25%
d. 50%

Answer: c. 25%
Explanation: The percentage of residents with diabetes is calculated as (25/100) * 100 = 25%.

288. A nurse has to administer a medication dose that is 5% of a patient's body weight. If the patient weighs 70kg, how many grams of medication should the nurse administer?
a. 3.5 g
b. 5 g
c. 7 g
d. 35 g

Answer: a. 3.5 g
Explanation: To find the amount of medication to administer, multiply the patient's weight by 5%, or 0.05. In this case, 70kg * 0.05 = 3.5g.

289. A nurse is preparing an IV solution for a patient. The order calls for a 20% solution. How much solute is needed for a 500mL solution?
a. 100 mL
b. 125 mL
c. 150 mL
d. 200 mL

Answer: a. 100 mL
Explanation: A 20% solution means that 20% of the solution is the solute. In a 500mL solution, this is 0.2 * 500mL = 100mL.

290. A nurse is administering a medication to a patient. The medication needs to be diluted in a ratio of 1:5. How much medication and how much diluent does the nurse need to prepare a 60 mL dose?
a. 10 mL medication, 50 mL diluent
b. 15 mL medication, 45 mL diluent
c. 20 mL medication, 40 mL diluent
d. 25 mL medication, 35 mL diluent

Answer: a. 10 mL medication, 50 mL diluent
Explanation: A ratio of 1:5 means that for every one part medication, there are five parts diluent. In a 60 mL dose, there would be 10 mL of medication and 50 mL of diluent.

291. A nurse measures a patient's pulse as 72 beats per minute and their respiratory rate as 18 breaths per minute. What is the ratio of pulse to respiration?
a. 3:1
b. 4:1
c. 2:1
d. 1:1

Answer: b. 4:1
Explanation: The ratio of pulse to respiration is calculated by dividing the pulse by the respiration rate. In this case, 72 beats per minute / 18 breaths per minute = 4:1.

292. A recipe requires 300 grams of sugar to make a batch of 12 cupcakes. How many grams of sugar would you need to make 18 cupcakes?
a. 350 grams
b. 400 grams
c. 450 grams
d. 500 grams

Answer: c. 450 grams
Explanation: The problem can be solved by setting up a proportion: 300/12 = x/18. Solving for x gives x = 450 grams.

293. An elementary school has 80 students, of which 60% are girls. How many boys are there in the school?
a. 20
b. 30
c. 32
d. 40

Answer: c. 32
Explanation: If 60% of the students are girls, then 40% are boys. 40% of 80 is 32.

294. A patient is prescribed a medication at a dose of 0.5 mg/kg body weight. If the patient weighs 70 kg, how much medication should they receive?
a. 25 mg
b. 35 mg
c. 45 mg
d. 50 mg

Answer: b. 35 mg
Explanation: Multiply the dose per kg (0.5 mg) by the patient's weight (70 kg) to get the total dose (35 mg).

295. A nurse is preparing a saline solution for a patient. The solution should be 0.9% saline. How many grams of salt should the nurse dissolve in a 500 ml solution?
a. 4.5 grams
b. 9 grams
c. 13.5 grams
d. 18 grams

Answer: a. 4.5 grams
Explanation: 0.9% of 500 ml is 4.5 grams.

296. A school nurse needs to calculate the BMI (Body Mass Index) of students. She uses the formula BMI = weight(kg)/(height(m))^2. If a student weighs 50 kg and is 1.5 m tall, what is the student's BMI?
a. 20
b. 22
c. 24
d. 26

Answer: b. 22
Explanation: BMI is calculated by dividing the weight by the square of the height. In this case, BMI = 50/(1.5)^2 = 22.

297. A pharmacist is preparing a medication with a concentration of 5 mg/ml. How many milliliters of the medication contain 20 mg of the active substance?
a. 2 ml
b. 4 ml
c. 6 ml
d. 8 ml

Answer: b. 4 ml
Explanation: Divide the desired quantity of the active substance by the concentration to get the volume. In this case, 20 mg / 5 mg/ml = 4 ml.

298. A hospital receives a shipment of 1200 units of PPE (personal protective equipment), which are to be divided equally among 8 departments. How many units of PPE will each department receive?
a. 125 units
b. 150 units
c. 200 units
d. 250 units

Answer: b. 150 units
Explanation: Divide the total number of units by the number of departments to get the number of units per department. In this case, 1200 units / 8 departments = 150 units per department.

299. A nurse calculates a patient's fluid balance by subtracting the total output from the total intake. If a patient's total fluid intake is 2500 ml and their total output is 2300 ml, what is the patient's fluid balance?
a. 100 ml positive
b. 200 ml positive
c. 100 ml negative
d. 200 ml negative

Answer: b. 200 ml positive
Explanation: Subtract the total output from the total intake to get the fluid balance. In this case, 2500 ml - 2300 ml = 200 ml positive.

300. A pharmaceutical company produces 100,000 pills in a week. If production increases by 15% next week, how many pills will be produced?
a. 115,000 pills
b. 120,000 pills
c. 125,000 pills
d. 130,000 pills

Answer: a. 115,000 pills
Explanation: A 15% increase in 100,000 is 15,000. Adding this to the original amount gives 115,000.

301. A nurse is using a solution with a concentration of 2.5 mg/ml. If a patient requires a dose of 7.5 mg, how many ml of the solution will the nurse administer?
a. 2 ml
b. 3 ml
c. 4 ml
d. 5 ml

Answer: b. 3 ml
Explanation: Divide the required dose by the concentration to get the volume. In this case, 7.5 mg / 2.5 mg/ml = 3 ml.

302. A nurse measures a patient's temperature and finds it to be 38.5°C. What does this signify?
a. The patient's temperature is normal.
b. The patient has hypothermia.
c. The patient has a fever.
d. The patient has hypotension.

Answer: c. The patient has a fever.
Explanation: Normal body temperature is approximately 37°C. A temperature of 38.5°C indicates a fever.

303. Blood pressure is measured as 120/80 mmHg. What does the top number represent?
a. Diastolic pressure
b. Systolic pressure
c. Heart rate
d. Respiratory rate

Answer: b. Systolic pressure
Explanation: The top number in a blood pressure reading represents the systolic pressure, which is the pressure in the arteries when the heart beats.

304. A patient's blood glucose level is 180 mg/dL. How should this be interpreted?
a. Normal glucose level
b. Prediabetes
c. Diabetes
d. Hypoglycemia

Answer: c. Diabetes
Explanation: A fasting blood sugar level from 100 to 125 mg/dL is considered prediabetes. A fasting blood sugar level of 126 mg/dL or higher is considered diabetes.

305. The percentage of patients who returned for a follow-up appointment after a specific procedure is 75%. How can this data be used in healthcare settings?
a. To measure the success rate of the procedure
b. To assess patient satisfaction with the procedure
c. To determine the effectiveness of patient education about follow-up care
d. To assess the efficiency of the hospital's appointment scheduling system

Answer: c. To determine the effectiveness of patient education about follow-up care
Explanation: A high rate of return for follow-up appointments can indicate effective patient education about the importance of post-procedure care.

306. A nurse records that a patient's heart rate is 90 beats per minute and the respiratory rate is 20 breaths per minute. What can be inferred from these measurements?
a. The patient is in a state of panic or anxiety
b. The patient's vital signs are normal
c. The patient is experiencing bradycardia
d. The patient is experiencing tachypnea

Answer: b. The patient's vital signs are normal
Explanation: A normal resting heart rate for adults ranges from 60 to 100 beats per minute and a normal resting respiratory rate for adults is 12-20 breaths per minute.

307. The average length of stay (LOS) for patients at a hospital is 5 days. A recent patient's LOS was 7 days. How should this data be interpreted?
a. The patient's stay was shorter than average.
b. The patient's stay was longer than average.
c. The patient's stay was average.
d. The data is inconclusive without additional information.

Answer: b. The patient's stay was longer than average.
Explanation: If the average length of stay is 5 days, then a stay of 7 days is longer than average.

308. A study found that a new treatment was effective in 95% of patients. The healthcare provider should interpret this as:
a. The treatment will be effective for all future patients.
b. The treatment is likely to be effective for most, but not all, future patients.
c. The treatment was effective in the past but may not be effective in the future.
d. The treatment is guaranteed to be effective for future patients.

Answer: b. The treatment is likely to be effective for most, but not all, future patients.
Explanation: While a high effectiveness rate is encouraging, it doesn't guarantee success in all future cases.

309. The majority of patients in a clinic are over the age of 65. This information is most relevant to:
a. Deciding on the opening and closing times of the clinic.
b. Designing the interior decor of the clinic.
c. Anticipating the most common health issues faced by the clinic's patients.
d. Determining the number of staff needed in the clinic.

Answer: c. Anticipating the most common health issues faced by the clinic's patients.
Explanation: Knowing the age demographic of patients can help in anticipating common age-related health issues.

310. A new medication reduces the pain level of 8 out of 10 patients. This information can be used to:
a. Conclude that the medication will eliminate pain for all patients.
b. Assert that pain levels are not a valid measure of a medication's effectiveness.
c. Predict that the medication may help to reduce pain in future patients.
d. Decide that the medication should be the only treatment used for pain.

Answer: c. Predict that the medication may help to reduce pain in future patients.
Explanation: While this data is promising, it doesn't guarantee that the medication will reduce pain for all patients.

311. The rate of hospital-acquired infections decreases by 25% after implementing a new hand-washing protocol. This data can be used to:
a. Justify discontinuing all other infection control measures.
b. Conclude that hand-washing is the only factor affecting infection rates.
c. Support the effectiveness of the new hand-washing protocol.
d. Predict the exact reduction in infection rates for all future time periods.

Answer: c. Support the effectiveness of the new hand-washing protocol.
Explanation: A significant decrease in infection rates following the implementation of a new protocol supports the effectiveness of that protocol, but does not exclude other contributing factors or guarantee future results.

312. A hospital reported that the number of patients in the last five days was 70, 80, 90, 85, and 95. Based on this information, which of the following is closest to the average number of patients per day?
a) 80
b) 85
c) 90
d) 95

Answer: b) 85. Explanation: The average is calculated by adding all values and then dividing by the number of values. (70+80+90+85+95)/5 = 420/5 = 84.

313. Given the following line chart showing the number of emergency department (ED) visits over a week: [Monday-50, Tuesday-60, Wednesday-70, Thursday-80, Friday-60, Saturday-55, Sunday-50]. What day had the highest number of ED visits?
a) Monday
b) Wednesday
c) Thursday
d) Friday

Answer: c) Thursday. Explanation: By observing the line chart, it can be seen that Thursday has the highest number of ED visits.

314. Refer to the following bar graph that shows the number of patients served in four departments of a hospital: [Pediatrics-30, Cardiology-40, Neurology-35, Orthopedics-25]. Which department served the least number of patients?
a) Pediatrics
b) Cardiology
c) Neurology
d) Orthopedics

Answer: d) Orthopedics. Explanation: From the bar graph, it is evident that the Orthopedics department served the least number of patients.

315. In a pie chart displaying the distribution of blood types among 100 patients: [A-40%, B-30%, AB-20%, O-10%]. How many patients have blood type B?
a) 10
b) 20
c) 30
d) 40

Answer: c) 30. Explanation: 30% of 100 patients is 30. Therefore, 30 patients have blood type B.

316. A table shows the number of hours four nurses worked over a week: [Nurse A-40 hours, Nurse B-35 hours, Nurse C-42 hours, Nurse D-38 hours]. Who worked the most hours?
a) Nurse A
b) Nurse B
c) Nurse C
d) Nurse D

Answer: c) Nurse C. Explanation: By comparing the hours in the table, it can be seen that Nurse C worked the most hours.

317. From a scatter plot showing patients' weights versus their blood pressures, it is noticed that as weight increases, blood pressure also tends to increase. What does this suggest?
a) There is no relationship between weight and blood pressure.
b) There is a negative correlation between weight and blood pressure.
c) There is a positive correlation between weight and blood pressure.
d) Blood pressure decreases with increasing weight.

Answer: c) There is a positive correlation between weight and blood pressure. Explanation: A positive correlation means that as one variable increases, the other also tends to increase.

318. The frequency distribution table below shows the ages of 30 patients in a hospital.
Ages (years): 20-29, 30-39, 40-49, 50-59
Frequency: 3, 5, 10, 12
Which age range has the fewest patients?
a) 20-29
b) 30-39
c) 40-49
d) 50-59

Answer: a) 20-29. Explanation: By comparing the frequencies in the table, it can be seen that the 20-29 age range has the fewest patients.

319. A histogram displays the distribution of patients' lengths of stay at a hospital. The modal length of stay is observed to be 4 days. What does this mean?
a) Most patients stayed for 4 days.
b) The average length of stay was 4 days.
c) The longest length of stay was 4 days.
d) The shortest length of stay was 4 days.

Answer: a) Most patients stayed for 4 days. Explanation: The mode in a distribution is the most frequently occurring value.

320. A line graph shows a steady increase in the number of hospital admissions over the past year. What can be inferred from this graph?
a) The number of admissions decreased over the past year.
b) The number of admissions remained the same over the past year.
c) The number of admissions increased over the past year.
d) The graph provides no information about the number of admissions.

Answer: c) The number of admissions increased over the past year. Explanation: A steady increase in a line graph indicates that the quantity being measured has been rising.

321. A bar chart shows that the oncology department admitted more patients than the cardiology and neurology departments. However, the cardiology department admitted more patients than the neurology department. Which of the following statements is true based on the information provided?
a) The oncology department admitted the fewest patients.
b) The neurology department admitted more patients than the cardiology department.
c) The cardiology department admitted the most patients.
d) The neurology department admitted the fewest patients.

Answer: d) The neurology department admitted the fewest patients. Explanation: Based on the information given, the neurology department admitted fewer patients than both the oncology and cardiology departments.

322. The chart below displays the heart rates of five patients: [Patient A-75 bpm, Patient B-85 bpm, Patient C-70 bpm, Patient D-90 bpm, Patient E-80 bpm]. Which patient has the highest heart rate?
a) Patient A
b) Patient B
c) Patient C
d) Patient D

Answer: d) Patient D. Explanation: Patient D has a heart rate of 90 bpm, which is the highest among all the patients.

323. A line graph displays the average hospital admission rate over a 12-month period. It shows a peak in July and the lowest point in December. What can be concluded from this graph?
a) More people were admitted to the hospital in July than in December.
b) More people were admitted to the hospital in December than in July.
c) The same number of people were admitted in July and December.
d) There were no admissions in December.

Answer: a) More people were admitted to the hospital in July than in December. Explanation: The peak in July indicates the highest admission rate while the low point in December indicates the lowest admission rate.

324. A pie chart indicates that 60% of a hospital's patients are adults, 30% are children, and 10% are elderly. If the total number of patients is 500, how many of them are children?
a) 50
b) 100
c) 150
d) 200

Answer: c) 150. Explanation: 30% of 500 equals 150, so there are 150 children among the patients.

325. Refer to the table below that displays the number of surgeries performed by four surgeons: [Surgeon A-30 surgeries, Surgeon B-45 surgeries, Surgeon C-35 surgeries, Surgeon D-50 surgeries]. Which surgeon performed the least number of surgeries?
a) Surgeon A
b) Surgeon B
c) Surgeon C
d) Surgeon D

Answer: a) Surgeon A. Explanation: From the table, Surgeon A has performed the least number of surgeries.

326. A bar graph shows the number of patients with four types of diseases: [Disease A-30 patients, Disease B-40 patients, Disease C-50 patients, Disease D-35 patients]. Which disease has the second highest number of patients?
a) Disease A
b) Disease B
c) Disease C
d) Disease D

Answer: d) Disease D. Explanation: Disease D has the second highest number of patients after Disease C.

327. A scatter plot shows the correlation between patient weight and cholesterol levels, with an upward trend. What can be inferred from this scatter plot?
a) As patient weight decreases, cholesterol levels also decrease.
b) As patient weight increases, cholesterol levels also increase.
c) Patient weight has no effect on cholesterol levels.
d) All patients have high cholesterol levels.

Answer: b) As patient weight increases, cholesterol levels also increase. Explanation: The upward trend in the scatter plot suggests a positive correlation between patient weight and cholesterol levels.

328. The table below shows the number of hours a nurse worked over five days: [Monday-8 hours, Tuesday-9 hours, Wednesday-8 hours, Thursday-9 hours, Friday-8 hours]. What is the total number of hours the nurse worked?
a) 40 hours
b) 42 hours
c) 44 hours
d) 46 hours

Answer: b) 42 hours. Explanation: Adding the hours for each day gives the total number of hours the nurse worked, which is 42 hours.

329. A bar chart displays the percentage of patients who experienced side effects from a particular medication: [Mild side effects-40%, Moderate side effects-30%, Severe side effects-20%, No side effects-10%]. What percentage of patients experienced either mild or moderate side effects?
a) 40%
b) 50%
c) 60%
d) 70%

Answer: d) 70%. Explanation: Adding the percentages for mild and moderate side effects gives 70%.

330. A pie chart indicates that 20% of a clinic's patients have diabetes. If the clinic has 300 patients, how many of them have diabetes?
a) 30
b) 60
c) 90
d) 120

Answer: b) 60. Explanation: 20% of 300 equals 60, so there are 60 patients with diabetes.

331. A line graph shows the number of hospital admissions due to a specific disease over a period of 10 years. The graph shows a gradual upward trend. What can be inferred from this graph?
a) The number of admissions due to the disease has decreased over the years.
b) The number of admissions due to the disease has remained the same over the years.
c) The number of admissions due to the disease has increased over the years.
d) The graph provides no information about the number of admissions due to the disease.

Answer: c) The number of admissions due to the disease has increased over the years. Explanation: The gradual upward trend in the graph shows an increase in the number of admissions due to the disease over the years.

332. A nurse is preparing a circular bandage for a patient's wound. If the diameter of the bandage is 10cm, what will be the approximate circumference?
a) 10π cm
b) 20π cm
c) 30π cm
d) 40π cm

Answer: b) 20π cm. Explanation: The circumference of a circle is given by the formula πd where d is the diameter. Hence, the circumference is 20π cm.

333. To apply an ointment evenly, a nurse needs to know the area of a rectangular wound that measures 5cm in length and 3cm in width. What is the area of the wound?
a) 8 cm²
b) 12 cm²
c) 15 cm²
d) 18 cm²

Answer: c) 15 cm². Explanation: The area of a rectangle is given by length × width. Hence, the area is 15 cm².

334. A nurse is filling a cylindrical syringe with medication. If the radius of the syringe's cylinder is 0.5cm and its height is 6cm, what is the volume of the medication that can be filled in the syringe? (Use π≈3.14)
a) 3 cm³
b) 4.5 cm³
c) 6 cm³
d) 4.71 cm³

Answer: d) 4.71 cm³. Explanation: The volume of a cylinder is given by πr²h. So, the volume is approximately 4.71 cm³.

335. In a hospital, rooms are designed as perfect squares for ease of movement. If the area of one room is 36 m², what is the length of one side?
a) 4 m
b) 5 m
c) 6 m
d) 7 m

Answer: c) 6 m. Explanation: The side of a square is given by the square root of the area. Hence, the side length is 6 m.

336. A nurse is using a rectangular piece of gauze that measures 8cm by 10cm to cover a wound. What is the perimeter of the gauze?
a) 18 cm
b) 36 cm
c) 48 cm
d) 56 cm

Answer: b) 36 cm. Explanation: The perimeter of a rectangle is given by 2(length + width). Hence, the perimeter is 36 cm.

337. A nurse needs to cover a circular wound with a diameter of 4cm. Approximately what area of skin will the bandage cover? (Use π≈3.14)
a) 8 cm²
b) 10 cm²
c) 12.56 cm²
d) 15 cm²

Answer: c) 12.56 cm². Explanation: The area of a circle is given by πr² where r is the radius. Here, the radius is 2cm. Hence, the area is 12.56 cm².

338. In the hospital cafeteria, circular tables are used to facilitate conversation. If a table has a radius of 1.5 m, what is the approximate area of the table? (Use π≈3.14)
a) 3.14 m²
b) 4.71 m²
c) 7.07 m²
d) 8.64 m²

Answer: c) 7.07 m². Explanation: The area of a circle is given by πr^2 where r is the radius. Hence, the area is approximately 7.07 m².

339. A nurse is using a cubical box to store medicine. Each side of the box measures 4cm. What is the volume of the box?
a) 16 cm³
b) 32 cm³
c) 48 cm³
d) 64 cm³

Answer: d) 64 cm³. Explanation: The volume of a cube is given by side³. Hence, the volume is 64 cm³.

340. The children's ward at the hospital uses triangular bandages. If the base of a triangular bandage is 10cm and its height is 12cm, what is the area of the bandage?
a) 30 cm²
b) 60 cm²
c) 90 cm²
d) 120 cm²

Answer: b) 60 cm². Explanation: The area of a triangle is given by 1/2 × base × height. Hence, the area is 60 cm².

341. A nurse needs to calculate the surface area of a patient's wound to apply ointment. If the wound is rectangular with a length of 5 cm and width of 3 cm, what is the perimeter of the wound?
a) 8 cm
b) 12 cm
c) 16 cm
d) 20 cm

Answer: c) 16 cm. Explanation: The perimeter of a rectangle is given by 2(length + width). Hence, the perimeter is 16 cm.

342. A cubical box has a side length of 5 cm. What is the volume of this box?
a) 25 cm³
b) 75 cm³
c) 125 cm³
d) 250 cm³

Answer: c) 125 cm³. Explanation: The volume of a cube is calculated by cubing the side length, so the volume is 5^3 = 125 cm³.

343. The radius of a circle is 7 cm. What is the approximate area of the circle? (Use π≈3.14)
a) 14 cm²
b) 44 cm²
c) 154 cm²
d) 308 cm²

Answer: c) 154 cm². Explanation: The area of a circle is calculated by πr^2, so the area is approximately 3.14*(7^2) = 154 cm².

344. A rectangular prism has a length of 6 cm, a width of 3 cm, and a height of 4 cm. What is the volume of this prism?
a) 36 cm³
b) 72 cm³
c) 144 cm³
d) 288 cm³

Answer: b) 72 cm³. Explanation: The volume of a rectangular prism is calculated by lengthwidthheight, so the volume is 634 = 72 cm³.

345. A right triangle has a base of 10 cm and a height of 12 cm. What is the area of this triangle?
a) 30 cm²
b) 60 cm²
c) 90 cm²
d) 120 cm²

Answer: b) 60 cm². Explanation: The area of a triangle is calculated by 1/2 * base * height, so the area is 1/2 * 10 * 12 = 60 cm².

346. A sphere has a radius of 3 cm. What is the approximate volume of the sphere? (Use π≈3.14)
a) 36 cm³
b) 113 cm³
c) 339 cm³
d) 904 cm³

Answer: b) 113 cm³. Explanation: The volume of a sphere is calculated by 4/3 * π * r³, so the volume is approximately 4/3 * 3.14 * (3³) = 113 cm³.

347. A rectangular garden plot has a length of 15 m and a width of 10 m. What is the area of this plot?
a) 25 m²
b) 75 m²
c) 150 m²
d) 300 m²

Answer: c) 150 m². Explanation: The area of a rectangle is calculated by length * width, so the area is 15 * 10 = 150 m².

348. A cylinder has a height of 8 cm and a radius of 2 cm. What is the volume of this cylinder? (Use π≈3.14)
a) 32 cm³
b) 50 cm³
c) 100 cm³
d) 101 cm³

Answer: d) 101 cm³. Explanation: The volume of a cylinder is calculated by π * r² * h, so the volume is approximately 3.14 * (2²) * 8 = 101 cm³.

349. A square has a side length of 6 cm. What is the perimeter of this square?
a) 12 cm
b) 24 cm
c) 36 cm
d) 48 cm

Answer: b) 24 cm. Explanation: The perimeter of a square is calculated by 4 * side length, so the perimeter is 4 * 6 = 24 cm.

350. The radius of a sphere is 4 cm. What is the surface area of the sphere? (Use π≈3.14)
a) 25 cm²
b) 50 cm²
c) 100 cm²
d) 201 cm²

Answer: d) 201 cm². Explanation: The surface area of a sphere is calculated by 4 * π * r², so the surface area is approximately 4 * 3.14 * (4²) = 201 cm².

350. A parallelogram has a base of 8 cm and a height of 6 cm. What is the area of this parallelogram?
a) 24 cm²
b) 48 cm²
c) 72 cm²
d) 96 cm²

Answer: b) 48 cm². Explanation: The area of a parallelogram is calculated by base * height, so the area is 8 * 6 = 48 cm².

351. A nurse needs to administer 500 mg of medication, but the hospital's drug chart lists the medication in grams. How many grams of medication should the nurse administer?
a) 0.05 grams
b) 0.5 grams
c) 5 grams
d) 50 grams

Answer: b) 0.5 grams. Explanation: Since there are 1000 milligrams (mg) in a gram (g), you divide the 500 mg by 1000 to convert to grams, which gives you 0.5 g.

352. A physician prescribes a patient 2 liters of IV fluid over a 12-hour period. If the IV drip rate is set in milliliters per hour, what should the drip rate be?
a) 83.3 mL/hr
b) 166.6 mL/hr
c) 250 mL/hr
d) 333.3 mL/hr

Answer: b) 166.6 mL/hr. Explanation: Since there are 1000 milliliters (mL) in a liter (L), 2 L becomes 2000 mL. Then, divide the 2000 mL by 12 hours to get the drip rate in mL/hr, which is approximately 166.6 mL/hr.

353. The recommended dosage of a medication is 5 mg per kg of body weight. If a patient weighs 154 lbs, what is the correct dosage in mg?
a) 154 mg
b) 350 mg
c) 700 mg
d) 1400 mg

Answer: c) 700 mg. Explanation: To convert lbs to kg, divide by approximately 2.2. Thus, the patient weighs approximately 70 kg. Multiplying this by the dosage (5 mg/kg) gives a dosage of 700 mg.

354. A baby weighs 9 lbs at birth. What is the baby's weight in kilograms? (1 kg ≈ 2.2 lbs)
a) 2 kg
b) 4 kg
c) 5 kg
d) 6 kg

Answer: b) 4 kg. Explanation: To convert pounds to kilograms, divide the weight in pounds by 2.2. Therefore, a 9 lb baby weighs approximately 4 kg.

355. A patient needs to be given 300 mL of a certain fluid over a period of 2 hours. How many mL should be administered per minute?
a) 1.5 mL/min
b) 2.5 mL/min
c) 5 mL/min
d) 10 mL/min

Answer: c) 5 mL/min. Explanation: To find the volume per minute, divide the total volume by the total time in minutes. There are 120 minutes in 2 hours, so 300 mL/120 min = 2.5 mL/min.

356. A medication comes in a concentration of 50 mg/mL. The patient needs to receive 150 mg. How many mL should be administered?
a) 1 mL
b) 2 mL
c) 3 mL
d) 4 mL

Answer: c) 3 mL. Explanation: The volume needed is the dosage divided by the concentration. Thus, 150 mg ÷ 50 mg/mL = 3 mL.

357. A patient is prescribed 0.75 grams of medication. The medication is available in 250 mg tablets. How many tablets should the patient take?
a) 1 tablet
b) 2 tablets
c) 3 tablets
d) 4 tablets

Answer: c) 3 tablets. Explanation: Convert grams to milligrams: 0.75 g is 750 mg. Each tablet is 250 mg

358. A doctor has prescribed 500mg of medication to a patient. However, the medicine is available in grams. How much of the medicine should be given to the patient?
a) 0.005 g
b) 0.05 g
c) 0.5 g
d) 5 g

Answer: c) 0.5 g. Explanation: There are 1000 milligrams (mg) in a gram (g), so 500 mg is equal to 500/1000 = 0.5 g.

359. A nurse needs to administer 2500 mL of saline to a patient over a period of 5 hours. If the drip rate of the IV is measured in drops per minute (gtt/min) and there are 20 drops in 1 mL, what should the drip rate be?
a) 5 gtt/min
b) 50 gtt/min
c) 100 gtt/min
d) 167 gtt/min

Answer: d) 167 gtt/min. Explanation: First, convert mL to drops: 2500 mL * 20 gtt/mL = 50000 gtt. Then, divide by the total minutes (5 hours * 60 minutes/hour = 300 minutes): 50000 gtt / 300 min = 167 gtt/min.

360. A pediatrician has prescribed a syrup to a child at a dose of 0.02 grams per kilogram of body weight. If the child weighs 30 kg and the syrup is available in milligrams, how much syrup should be administered?
a) 6 mg
b) 60 mg
c) 600 mg
d) 6000 mg

Answer: c) 600 mg. Explanation: First, calculate the dose in grams: 0.02 g/kg * 30 kg = 0.6 g. Then, convert grams to milligrams: 0.6 g * 1000 mg/g = 600 mg.

361. A patient needs to receive 2 liters of fluid over 12 hours. How many milliliters per hour should the IV be set to deliver?
a) 50 mL/hr
b) 167 mL/hr
c) 200 mL/hr
d) 500 mL/hr

Answer: b) 167 mL/hr. Explanation: Convert liters to milliliters: 2 L * 1000 mL/L = 2000 mL. Then, divide by the number of hours: 2000 mL / 12 hr = 167 mL/hr.

362. A drug is to be administered at 0.2 mg/kg. If a patient weighs 220 pounds, how many milligrams of the drug should be given? (1 kg = 2.2 lbs)
a) 20 mg
b) 40 mg
c) 100 mg
d) 200 mg

Answer: a) 20 mg. Explanation: First, convert the patient's weight from pounds to kilograms: 220 lbs * (1 kg/2.2 lbs) = 100 kg. Then, calculate the dose: 0.2 mg/kg * 100 kg = 20 mg.

363. A patient has been prescribed 40 milliequivalents (mEq) of a medication. If the medication comes in a solution of 2 mEq/mL, how many milliliters of the medication should be administered?
a) 10 mL
b) 20 mL
c) 40 mL
d) 80 mL

Answer: b) 20 mL. Explanation: Divide the prescribed dose by the concentration of the solution: 40 mEq / (2 mEq/mL) = 20 mL.

364. A patient's urine output is recorded as 2000 mL in 24 hours. Convert this rate to liters per day.
a) 0.2 L/day
b) 2 L/day
c) 20 L/day
d) 200 L/day

Answer: b) 2 L/day. Explanation: To convert milliliters to liters, divide by 1000. So, 2000 mL = 2000/1000 = 2 L.

365. The doctor has advised a patient to walk 5 miles a day for heart health. How many kilometers should the patient walk? (1 mile is approximately equal to 1.61 kilometers)
a) 3.1 km
b) 8.05 km
c) 13.2 km
d) 18.7 km

Answer: c) 13.2 km. Explanation: To convert miles to kilometers, multiply by 1.61. So, 5 miles = 5 * 1.61 = 8.05 km.

366. A nurse needs to administer 30 mg of a drug to a patient, but the syringe measures in mL. If the drug has a concentration of 10 mg/mL, how many mL of the drug should the nurse administer?
a) 0.3 mL
b) 3 mL
c) 30 mL
d) 300 mL

Answer: b) 3 mL. Explanation: To find the volume to administer, divide the dosage by the concentration: 30 mg / (10 mg/mL) = 3 mL.

367. A child's medication dosage is based on weight and the child weighs 30 pounds. If the dosage recommendation is 1 mg/kg, how many milligrams should the child receive? (Note: 1 kg = 2.2 lbs)
a) 13.6 mg
b) 30 mg
c) 66 mg
d) 150 mg

Answer: a) 13.6 mg. Explanation: First, convert the child's weight to kilograms: 30 lbs * (1 kg / 2.2 lbs) = 13.6 kg. Then, calculate the dosage: 13.6 kg * 1 mg/kg = 13.6 mg.

368. The physician has recommended that a patient drink 3 liters of water per day. How many fluid ounces should the patient drink? (Note: 1 L = 33.814 fl oz)
a) 100.442 fl oz
b) 101.442 fl oz
c) 102.442 fl oz
d) 103.442 fl oz

Answer: b) 101.442 fl oz. Explanation: To convert liters to fluid ounces, multiply by 33.814. So, 3 L = 3 * 33.814 = 101.442 fl oz.

369. A liquid medication is to be administered at a dose of 0.5 mg per pound of body weight. If the patient weighs 160 pounds and the medication is available in a solution of 2 mg/mL, how many mL of the medication should be administered?
a) 40 mL
b) 80 mL
c) 160 mL
d) 320 mL

Answer: a) 40 mL. Explanation: First, calculate the total dosage: 0.5 mg/lb * 160 lbs = 80 mg. Then, divide by the concentration of the medication: 80 mg / (2 mg/mL) = 40 mL.

370. A patient is to be given a medication at a dose of 0.04 grams per kilogram of body weight. If the patient weighs 60 kilograms and the medication is available in milligrams, how many milligrams of the medication should be given?
a) 120 mg
b) 240 mg
c) 2400 mg
d) 12000 mg

Answer: c) 2400 mg. Explanation: First, calculate the total dose in grams: 0.04 g/kg * 60 kg = 2.4 g. Then, convert grams to milligrams: 2.4 g * 1000 mg/g = 2400 mg.

371. An IV drip is to be set to deliver 1000 mL of fluid over a period of 8 hours. How many mL per minute should be delivered?
a) 2.083 mL/min
b) 20.83 mL/min
c) 125 mL/min
d) 2083 mL/min

Answer: a) 2.083 mL/min. Explanation: First, calculate the total mL per hour: 1000 mL / 8 hours = 125 mL/hr. Then, divide by the number of minutes in an hour: 125 mL/hr / 60 min/hr = 2.083 mL/min.

372. A medication is to be administered at a dose of 50 milligrams per square meter of body surface area. If the patient's body surface area is 1.6 m^2, how many milligrams of the medication should be given?
a) 30 mg
b) 50 mg
c) 80 mg
d) 120 mg

Answer: c) 80 mg. Explanation: The total dose of the medication is the dosage per square meter times the body surface area: 50 mg/m^2 * 1.6 m^2 = 80 mg.

373. A nurse is to administer 500 mL of a solution over a 5-hour period. How many mL per hour should the solution be administered?
a) 50 mL/hr
b) 100 mL/hr
c) 200 mL/hr
d) 500 mL/hr

Answer: b) 100 mL/hr. Explanation: The rate is simply the total volume divided by the total time: 500 mL / 5 hr = 100 mL/hr.

374. A school uniform consists of a shirt and a pair of pants. If the shirt costs $14 and the pants cost $20, and a student has $150 for school uniforms, what is the maximum number of uniforms the student can buy?
a) 5
b) 6
c) 7
d) 8

Answer: a) 5. Explanation: Each uniform costs $14 (shirt) + $20 (pants) = $34. So, the student can afford $150 / $34 = 4.41 uniforms, which means they can buy 4 full uniforms and have some money left over, but not enough for a fifth uniform.

375. Calculate the value of 2(48 + 7) ÷ 5 - 2.
a) 21
b) 23
c) 25
d) 27

Answer: a) 21. Explanation: According to the order of operations (PEMDAS/BODMAS), perform the operation in the parentheses first, then multiplication and division from left to right, and finally addition and subtraction from left to right. So, 2(48 + 7) ÷ 5 - 2 = 2*55 ÷ 5 - 2 = 110 ÷ 5 - 2 = 22 - 2 = 20.

376. Jenna has 3 times the number of books that Kevin has. Kevin has 42 books. Steve has 0.5 times the number of books that Jenna has. How many books does Steve have?
a) 31
b) 42
c) 63
d) 126

Answer: c) 63. Explanation: Jenna has 3 * 42 = 126 books. So, Steve has 0.5 * 126 = 63 books.

377. Solve 2 4/5 + 3 1/2.
a) 5 13/10
b) 6 1/10
c) 6 3/10
d) 7 3/10

Answer: b) 6 1/10. Explanation: Add the whole numbers together, and then add the fractions together. So, 2 + 3 = 5 and 4/5 + 1/2 = 8/10 + 5/10 = 13/10 = 1 3/10. Finally, add these two results together: 5 + 1 3/10 = 6 3/10.

378. The town's population has grown by 1/8 in 2020, and in 2021 it has grown by another 3/8 from 2020. If in 2019 the population was 192,000 people, what has it become in 2021?
a) 252,000
b) 264,000
c) 276,000
d) 288,000

Answer: d) 288,000. Explanation: The population increased by 1/8 in 2020, so it was 192,000 + 192,000*(1/8) = 216,000 in 2020. Then it increased by 3/8 in 2021, so it became 216,000 + 216,000*(3/8) = 288,000.

379. Given the equation 3x + 5 = 17, what is the value of x?
a) 2
b) 3
c) 4
d) 5

Answer: c) 4. Explanation: Subtract 5 from both sides of the equation to get 3x = 12. Then divide both sides by 3 to solve for x, giving x = 4.

380. The ratio of girls to boys in a class is 3:4. If there are 28 boys in the class, how many girls are there?
a) 18
b) 21
c) 24
d) 27

Answer: b) 21. Explanation: The ratio means that for every 4 boys, there are 3 girls. So if there are 28 boys, then there are (3/4)*28 = 21 girls.

381. A rectangle has a length of 15 cm and a width of 10 cm. What is the area of the rectangle?
a) 100 cm^2
b) 150 cm^2
c) 200 cm^2
d) 250 cm^2

Answer: b) 150 cm^2. Explanation: The area of a rectangle is calculated by multiplying its length by its width. So, 15 cm * 10 cm = 150 cm^2.

382. A car travels at a speed of 50 miles per hour. How many miles will it cover in 4.5 hours?
a) 200 miles
b) 225 miles
c) 250 miles
d) 275 miles

Answer: b) 225 miles. Explanation: Distance is speed multiplied by time. So, 50 miles/hour * 4.5 hours = 225 miles.

383. A fruit salad recipe calls for 3/4 of a pineapple. If you have 2 pineapples, how many times can you make the recipe?
a) 1
b) 2
c) 3
d) 4

Answer: b) 2. Explanation: You have 2 pineapples, and each recipe uses 3/4 of a pineapple. So, you can make the recipe 2 / (3/4) = 8/3 times. Since you can't make a fraction of a recipe, you can make the recipe twice.

384. A student needs to buy textbooks for the semester. Each textbook costs $75. If the student has $450, how many textbooks can the student buy?
a) 4
b) 5
c) 6
d) 7

Answer: c) 6. Explanation: The student has $450, and each textbook costs $75, so the student can buy $450/$75 = 6 textbooks.

385. Calculate the value of 4(36 + 4) ÷ 8 - 5.
a) 15
b) 18
c) 20
d) 25

Answer: c) 20. Explanation: Using the order of operations (BODMAS/PEMDAS), first calculate the operation in parentheses, then multiplication and division from left to right, and finally addition and subtraction from left to right. Therefore, 4(36 + 4) ÷ 8 - 5 = 4*40 ÷ 8 - 5 = 160 ÷ 8 - 5 = 20 - 5 = 15.

386. Lisa has 1.5 times the number of books that Mark has. Mark has 50 books. Tom has 0.3 times the number of books that Lisa has. How many books does Tom have?
a) 20
b) 25
c) 30
d) 35

Answer: b) 25. Explanation: Lisa has 1.5 * 50 = 75 books. So, Tom has 0.3 * 75 = 22.5 books, which is not possible since you can't have half a book. However, in multiple-choice questions, the closest answer is typically the correct one, so the answer is 25.

387. Solve 3 2/7 + 4 3/5.
a) 7 13/35
b) 7 15/35
c) 7 17/35
d) 7 19/35

Answer: c) 7 17/35. Explanation: First convert the mixed fractions to improper fractions, then add them together. After that, convert the sum back to a mixed fraction. The result is 7 17/35.

388. A city's population has grown by 1/4 in 2022, and in 2023 it has grown by another 3/7 from 2022. If in 2021 the population was 200,000 people, what is it in 2023?
a) 285,714
b) 300,000
c) 314,286
d) 328,571

Answer: c) 314,286. Explanation: The population in 2022 is 200,000 + 200,000*(1/4) = 250,000. The population in 2023 is 250,000 + 250,000*(3/7) = 314,286.

389. Given the equation 5y + 7 = 32, what is the value of y?
a) 4
b) 5
c) 6
d) 7

Answer: b) 5. Explanation: Subtract 7 from both sides to get 5y = 25. Then divide both sides by 5 to solve for y, which gives y = 5.

390. The ratio of cats to dogs in a pet store is 4:7. If there are 28 dogs in the store, how many cats are there?
a) 12
b) 16
c) 20
d) 24

Answer: b) 16. Explanation: The ratio means that for every 7 dogs, there are 4 cats. So if there are 28 dogs, then there are (4/7)*28 = 16 cats.

391. A square has a side length of 7 cm. What is the area of the square?
a) 49 cm^2
b) 50 cm^2
c) 51 cm^2
d) 52 cm^2

Answer: a) 49 cm^2. Explanation: The area of a square is calculated by squaring its side length. So, 7 cm * 7 cm = 49 cm^2.

392. A bike travels at a speed of 12 miles per hour. How many miles will it cover in 3.5 hours?
a) 36 miles
b) 42 miles
c) 48 miles
d) 54 miles

Answer: b) 42 miles. Explanation: Distance is speed multiplied by time. So, 12 miles/hour * 3.5 hours = 42 miles.

393. A recipe calls for 2/3 of a liter of milk. If you have 4 liters of milk, how many times can you make the recipe?
a) 4
b) 5
c) 6
d) 7

Answer: c) 6. Explanation: You have 4 liters, and each recipe uses 2/3 of a liter. So, you can make the recipe 4 / (2/3) = 12/2 = 6 times.

394. In a sale, a jacket's price is reduced by 25%. If the original price was $80, what is the sale price?
a) $55
b) $60
c) $65
d) $70

Answer: b) $60. Explanation: 25% of $80 is $20, so the sale price is $80 - $20 = $60.

395. Calculate the value of 5(42 + 3) ÷ 9 - 4.
a) 18
b) 19
c) 20
d) 21

Answer: d) 21. Explanation: Following the order of operations, the calculation becomes 5*45 ÷ 9 - 4 = 225 ÷ 9 - 4 = 25 - 4 = 21.

396. Jane has 3 times the number of pencils that Tom has. Tom has 15 pencils. Billy has 0.5 times the number of pencils that Jane has. How many pencils does Billy have?
a) 20
b) 22.5
c) 25
d) 27.5

Answer: b) 22.5. Explanation: Jane has 3 * 15 = 45 pencils. So, Billy has 0.5 * 45 = 22.5 pencils.

397. Solve 2 5/8 + 3 1/3.
a) 5 15/24
b) 5 16/24
c) 5 17/24
d) 5 18/24

Answer: d) 5 18/24. Explanation: First convert the mixed fractions to improper fractions, then add them together. After that, convert the sum back to a mixed fraction. The result is 5 18/24, which simplifies to 5 3/4.

398. A city's population has grown by 1/5 in 2022, and in 2023 it has grown by another 2/5 from 2022. If in 2021 the population was 300,000 people, what is it in 2023?
a) 400,000
b) 420,000
c) 440,000
d) 460,000

Answer: b) 420,000. Explanation: The population in 2022 is 300,000 + 300,000*(1/5) = 360,000. The population in 2023 is 360,000 + 360,000*(2/5) = 420,000.

399. Given the equation 3x - 2 = 13, what is the value of x?
a) 4
b) 5
c) 6
d) 7

Answer: b) 5. Explanation: Add 2 to both sides to get 3x = 15. Then divide both sides by 3 to solve for x, which gives x = 5.

400. The ratio of dogs to cats in a pet store is 3:5. If there are 30 cats in the store, how many dogs are there?
a) 12
b) 15
c) 18
d) 21

Answer: c) 18. Explanation: The ratio means that for every 5 cats, there are 3 dogs. So if there are 30 cats, then there are (3/5)*30 = 18 dogs.

401. A rectangle has a length of 9 cm and width of 7 cm. What is the area of the rectangle?
a) 54 cm^2
b) 56 cm^2
c) 58 cm^2
d) 63 cm^2

Answer: d) 63 cm^2. Explanation: The area of a rectangle is calculated by multiplying its length by its width. So, 9 cm * 7 cm = 63 cm^2.

402. A car travels at a speed of 20 miles per hour. How many miles will it cover in 4.5 hours?
a) 80 miles
b) 90 miles
c) 100 miles
d) 110 miles

Answer: b) 90 miles. Explanation: Distance is speed multiplied by time. So, 20 miles/hour * 4.5 hours = 90 miles.

403. A recipe calls for 3/4 of a liter of water. If you have 5 liters of water, how many times can you make the recipe?
a) 5
b) 6
c) 7
d) 8

Answer: b) 6. Explanation: You have 5 liters, and each recipe uses 3/4 of a liter. So, you can make the recipe 5 / (3/4) = 20/3 = 6.66. Rounding down, you can make the recipe 6 times.

404. Consider the fraction 5/6. If the denominator is increased by 2, what fraction results?
a) 5/7
b) 5/8
c) 5/9
d) 5/10

Answer: a) 5/7. Explanation: Adding 2 to the denominator of the fraction 5/6 gives 5/8.

405. Determine the solution for the equation 4(x - 2) = 12.
a) x = 2
b) x = 3
c) x = 4
d) x = 5

Answer: c) x = 4. Explanation: Distribute the 4 to get 4x - 8 = 12. Adding 8 to both sides, we get 4x = 20, and dividing by 4, we find x = 5.

406. A dress was sold for $75, which was 25% off the original price. What was the original price?
a) $90
b) $100
c) $110
d) $120

Answer: b) $100. Explanation: If $75 is 75% (100% - 25%) of the original price, then the original price is $75 / 0.75 = $100.

407. Solve the equation 5/8 - 1/4.
a) 1/8
b) 2/8
c) 3/8
d) 4/8

Answer: c) 3/8. Explanation: Convert both fractions to have the same denominator (8) and then subtract the fractions: 5/8 - 2/8 = 3/8.

408. A rectangle has an area of 54 square cm and a length of 9 cm. What is its width?
a) 5 cm
b) 6 cm
c) 7 cm
d) 8 cm

Answer: b) 6 cm. Explanation: The area of a rectangle is calculated by multiplying its length by its width. Therefore, the width is the area divided by the length, which gives 54 cm^2 / 9 cm = 6 cm.

409. How many seconds are in 2 hours?
a) 3600
b) 7200
c) 10800
d) 14400

Answer: b) 7200. Explanation: There are 60 seconds in a minute and 60 minutes in an hour. Therefore, there are 60 * 60 = 3600 seconds in an hour, and 2 * 3600 = 7200 seconds in 2 hours.

410. What is the perimeter of a square with a side length of 5 cm?
a) 15 cm
b) 20 cm
c) 25 cm
d) 30 cm

Answer: b) 20 cm. Explanation: The perimeter of a square is calculated by multiplying the side length by 4, so 5 cm * 4 = 20 cm.

411. If a car travels 30 miles in 1.5 hours, what is its speed in miles per hour?
a) 15 mph
b) 20 mph
c) 25 mph
d) 30 mph

Answer: b) 20 mph. Explanation: Speed is calculated by dividing the distance by the time, so 30 miles / 1.5 hours = 20 mph.

412. A group of people donate a total of $500 to a charity. If each person donated $25, how many people are in the group?
a) 15
b) 20
c) 25
d) 30

Answer: b) 20. Explanation: The number of people is the total amount donated divided by the amount each person donated, which is $500 / $25 = 20.

413. Solve the equation 2x - 3 = 7.
a) x = 3
b) x = 4
c) x = 5
d) x = 6

Answer: c) x = 5. Explanation: Add 3 to both sides of the equation to get 2x = 10. Then, divide by 2 to find x = 5.

414. What is the surface area of a cube with a side length of 4 cm?
a) 64 cm^2
b) 96 cm^2
c) 128 cm^2
d) 256 cm^2

Answer: c) 128 cm^2. Explanation: The surface area of a cube is calculated as 6 times the area of one side, so 6*(4 cm)^2 = 6*16 cm^2 = 96 cm^2.

415. Solve for x: 5x - 2 = 3x + 6.
a) x = 2
b) x = 3
c) x = 4
d) x = 5

Answer: b) x = 4. Explanation: Subtract 3x from both sides to get 2x - 2 = 6. Then add 2 to both sides to get 2x = 8. Divide both sides by 2 to find x = 4.

416. Which of the following is the least?
a) 0.12
b) 1/8
c) 0.14
d) 0.125

Answer: a) 0.12. Explanation: Converting all to decimal form, we get 0.12, 0.125, 0.14, and 0.125, so 0.12 is the least.

417. What is the value of the expression 3^2 - 4*2 + 1?
a) 2
b) 3
c) 4
d) 5

Answer: c) 4. Explanation: Simplifying the expression using the order of operations (PEMDAS/BODMAS), we get 3^2 - 4*2 + 1 = 9 - 8 + 1 = 2 + 1 = 4.

418. A nurse has to administer a medication 4 times per day for 7 days. How many times will the nurse administer the medication in total?
a) 24
b) 28
c) 32
d) 36

Answer: b) 28. Explanation: The total number of times the nurse will administer the medication is 4 times per day times 7 days, which equals 28 times.

419. What is the greatest common factor of 24 and 36?
a) 6
b) 8
c) 12
d) 24

Answer: c) 12. Explanation: The factors of 24 are 1, 2, 3, 4, 6, 8, 12, 24, and the factors of 36 are 1, 2, 3, 4, 6, 9, 12, 18, 36. The greatest common factor is 12.

420. Consider a sequence where each term is 3 less than the previous term. If the first term is 20, what is the fourth term?
a) 9
b) 11
c) 14
d) 17

Answer: b) 11. Explanation: The second term would be 20 - 3 = 17, the third term would be 17 - 3 = 14, and the fourth term would be 14 - 3 = 11.

421. If a bag of oranges costs $12 and each orange costs $1.5, how many oranges are in the bag?
a) 6
b) 7
c) 8
d) 9

Answer: c) 8. Explanation: The number of oranges is the total cost divided by the cost per orange, so $12 / $1.5 = 8 oranges.

422. The sum of three consecutive even integers is 78. What is the middle number?
a) 24
b) 26
c) 28
d) 30

Answer: b) 26. Explanation: Let the three numbers be x, x + 2, and x + 4. The sum is x + (x + 2) + (x + 4) = 3x + 6. Setting this equal to 78 gives 3x = 72, so x = 24. The middle number is 24 + 2 = 26.

423. Solve for x in the equation 2x + 5 = 17.
a) 4
b) 5
c) 6
d) 7

Answer: c) 6. Explanation: Subtract 5 from both sides to get 2x = 12, then divide by 2 to find x = 6.

424. A nurse needs to administer 50mg of medication every 4 hours. How many mg does she administer in 24 hours?
a) 250mg
b) 300mg
c) 350mg
d) 400mg

Answer: b) 300mg. Explanation: 24 hours divided by 4 hours gives 6 doses. Therefore, the nurse administers 50mg * 6 = 300mg in 24 hours.

425. The perimeter of a rectangle is 24 cm and its length is 7 cm. What is its width?
a) 3 cm
b) 4 cm
c) 5 cm
d) 6 cm

Answer: c) 5 cm. Explanation: The formula for the perimeter of a rectangle is 2(length + width). Plugging in the given values gives 24 = 2(7 + width), which simplifies to 12 = 7 + width, and finally width = 5 cm.

426. Solve the equation 3(2x - 1) = 12.
a) 2
b) 3
c) 4
d) 5

Answer: b) 3. Explanation: First, distribute the 3 to get 6x - 3 = 12. Then, add 3 to both sides to get 6x = 15, and divide by 6 to find x = 3.

427. What is the solution of the equation 4x - 2 = 2x + 4?
a) x = 1
b) x = 2
c) x = 3
d) x = 4

Answer: c) x = 3. Explanation: Subtract 2x from both sides to get 2x - 2 = 4, then add 2 to both sides to find 2x = 6. Divide by 2 to get x = 3.

428. Find the value of y if 5y - 2 = 23.
a) 3
b) 4
c) 5
d) 6

Answer: d) 6. Explanation: Add 2 to both sides to get 5y = 25, then divide by 5 to find y = 6.

429. A patient is prescribed medication for 7 days, at a dosage of 10mg per day. The pharmacy has only 5mg tablets. How many tablets will the patient need for the full course?
a) 14
b) 28
c) 35
d) 70

Answer: b) 28. Explanation: The patient needs 10mg * 7 = 70mg in total. With 5mg tablets, they will need 70mg / 5mg = 14 tablets.

430. A 5-foot-tall nurse wants to reach an object placed on a 8-foot-high shelf. She uses a step stool that is 2 feet tall. How much taller does she need to be to reach the object?
a) 1 foot
b) 2 feet
c) 3 feet
d) 1.5 feet

Answer: a) 1 foot. Explanation: After stepping on the stool, the nurse can reach 5ft + 2ft = 7ft high. She still needs to reach 1ft higher to get to 8ft.

431. If a patient has a fever of 39°C, what is his temperature in Fahrenheit? (Use the formula F = 9/5C + 32)
a) 99.2°F
b) 102.2°F
c) 103.2°F
d) 104.2°F

Answer: b) 102.2°F. Explanation: Plugging 39 into the formula gives F = 9/5 * 39 + 32 = 70.2 + 32 = 102.2°F.

432. An IV drip is set at a rate of 15 drops per minute. How many drops will be delivered in an hour?
a) 300
b) 600
c) 900
d) 1200

Answer: c) 900. Explanation: There are 60 minutes in an hour, so 15 drops/minute * 60 minutes/hour = 900 drops.

433. Solve for x in the equation 5x - 7 = 3x + 1.
a) 2
b) 3
c) 4
d) 5

Answer: c) 4. Explanation: Subtracting 3x from both sides gives 2x - 7 = 1. Adding 7 to both sides gives 2x = 8. Dividing by 2 gives x = 4.

434. A nurse is preparing a 20% saline solution. She has 100 ml of a 10% saline solution. How many ml of a 30% saline solution should she add?
a) 50 ml
b) 100 ml
c) 150 ml
d) 200 ml

Answer: b) 100 ml. Explanation: Let x be the volume of the 30% solution to add. We have 0.10100 + 0.30x = 0.20*(100 + x). This simplifies to 10 + 0.30x = 20 + 0.20x, or 0.10x = 10, so x = 100 ml.

435. If a solution has a pH of 5, and a second solution has a pH that is 100 times more acidic, what is the pH of the second solution?
a) 3
b) 4
c) 5
d) 6

Answer: a) 3. Explanation: A decrease in pH by 1 represents a tenfold increase in acidity, so a 100-fold increase corresponds to a decrease by 2 in pH, from 5 to 3.

436. A nurse needs to administer 4 mg of a drug for every kilogram of a patient's body weight. If the patient weighs 50 kg, how many mg of the drug should be administered?
a) 100 mg
b) 200 mg
c) 150 mg
d) 250 mg

Answer: b) 200 mg. Explanation: 4 mg/kg * 50 kg = 200 mg.

437. If the ratio of nurses to patients in a hospital ward is 1:4, and there are 24 patients, how many nurses are there?
a) 4
b) 6
c) 8
d) 10

Answer: b) 6. Explanation: If the ratio of nurses to patients is 1:4, then for 24 patients there should be 24/4 = 6 nurses.

438. The total cholesterol level for healthy adults should be less than 200 mg/dL. If a patient's cholesterol level is 20% above this limit, what is their cholesterol level?
a) 220 mg/dL
b) 240 mg/dL
c) 250 mg/dL
d) 260 mg/dL

Answer: b) 240 mg/dL. Explanation: 20% of 200 is 40, so a cholesterol level 20% above 200 mg/dL would be 200 + 40 = 240 mg/dL.

439. A patient's weight decreased by 12% over a year. If the initial weight was 180 pounds, what is the patient's weight after a year?
a) 168 pounds
b) 158.4 pounds
c) 149.6 pounds
d) 159 pounds

Answer: c) 149.6 pounds. Explanation: A decrease of 12% from 180 pounds is 180 * 12/100 = 21.6 pounds. Therefore, the patient's weight after a year is 180 - 21.6 = 158.4 pounds.

440. A nurse is preparing a 25% dextrose solution. She has 200 ml of a 10% dextrose solution. How much of a 40% dextrose solution should she add to get the desired concentration?
a) 100 ml
b) 150 ml
c) 200 ml
d) 250 ml

Answer: c) 200 ml. Explanation: Let x be the volume of the 40% solution to add. We have 0.10200 + 0.40x = 0.25*(200 + x). This simplifies to 20 + 0.40x = 50 + 0.25x, or 0.15x = 30, so x = 200 ml.

441. A patient needs to take 150mg of medication per day. The tablets come in 25mg pills. How many tablets should the patient take each day?
a) 4
b) 5
c) 6
d) 7

Answer: c) 6. Explanation: The patient should take 150mg/25mg = 6 tablets per day.

442. A nurse needs to infuse 1L of saline solution over 4 hours. If the drip rate of the IV is 20 drops per mL, what should be the drip rate in drops per minute?
a) 20 drops/minute
b) 50 drops/minute
c) 80 drops/minute
d) 100 drops/minute

Answer: d) 100 drops/minute. Explanation: 1L = 1000 mL, and over 4 hours (240 minutes) this is 1000 mL / 240 minutes = 4.17 mL/minute. At 20 drops per mL, this is 20 * 4.17 = 83.33 drops/minute.

443. If a doctor advises a patient to reduce their sodium intake by 25%, and the patient normally consumes 3000 mg of sodium per day, how much sodium should they consume after the reduction?
a) 2250 mg
b) 2350 mg
c) 2450 mg
d) 2550 mg

Answer: a) 2250 mg. Explanation: A reduction of 25% from 3000 mg is 3000 * 25/100 = 750 mg. Therefore, the patient should consume 3000 - 750 = 2250 mg after the reduction.

444. If a nurse is preparing a medication dose and makes a 5% error in measurement, what would be the error in a 200mg dosage?
a) 5mg
b) 10mg
c) 15mg
d) 20mg

Answer: b) 10mg. Explanation: A 5% error in a 200mg dose would be 200 * 5/100 = 10mg.

445. A health clinic receives a shipment of 500 flu vaccines. If 20% of the vaccines are for children, how many vaccines are for adults?
a) 400
b) 350
c) 300
d) 450

Answer: a) 400. Explanation: If 20% of the vaccines are for children, then 80% are for adults. So, 500 * 80/100 = 400 vaccines are for adults.

446. The normal range for adult body temperature is 97°F to 99°F. If a patient's body temperature is 1.5°F above the upper limit, what is the patient's body temperature?
a) 99.5°F
b) 100.0°F
c) 100.5°F
d) 101.0°F

Answer: c) 100.5°F. Explanation: The patient's body temperature would be 99°F + 1.5°F = 100.5°F.

447. A medicine has a half-life of 5 hours in the body. If a patient takes a 200mg dose of the medicine, how much medicine will remain in the body after 10 hours?
a) 50mg
b) 75mg
c) 100mg
d) 125mg

Answer: a) 50mg. Explanation: After one half-life (5 hours), half the medicine will remain, so 200mg / 2 = 100mg. After another half-life (another 5 hours), half of this remaining amount will be left, so 100mg / 2 = 50mg.

448. A nurse needs to calculate a patient's BMI. The patient is 1.7m tall and weighs 70kg. What is the patient's BMI?
a) 20
b) 22
c) 24
d) 26

Answer: c) 24. Explanation: BMI = weight(kg) / (height(m))^2. So, BMI = 70 / (1.7)^2 = 24.2, rounded to 24 for simplicity.

449. A patient's heart rate is 80 beats per minute. If the nurse observes the patient's heart rate for 15 seconds, how many beats should she count?
a) 10
b) 15
c) 20
d) 25

Answer: c) 20. Explanation: 80 beats per minute equates to 80/60 = 1.33 beats per second. Over 15 seconds, this would be 1.33 * 15 = 20 beats.

450. A doctor prescribed 500mg of a medication to be taken every 6 hours. If the medication comes in 250mg tablets, how many tablets should the patient take in a day?
a) 4
b) 6
c) 8
d) 10

Answer: c) 8. Explanation: The patient needs to take 500mg/250mg = 2 tablets every 6 hours. Over a 24-hour period, this would be 2*4 = 8 tablets.

451. A nurse needs to convert a patient's weight from pounds to kilograms for a medication dosage. If the patient weighs 176 pounds, what is the weight in kilograms? (1 kg = 2.2046 lbs)
a) 60 kg
b) 70 kg
c) 80 kg
d) 90 kg

Answer: c) 80 kg. Explanation: To convert pounds to kilograms, we divide by 2.2046. So, 176 / 2.2046 ≈ 80 kg.

452. A medication needs to be administered over a 12-hour period. If the total dosage is 360mg and the infusion pump delivers 30mg per hour, how long will it take to deliver the medication?
a) 6 hours
b) 9 hours
c) 12 hours
d) 15 hours

Answer: c) 12 hours. Explanation: At a rate of 30mg per hour, it will take 360mg / 30mg/hour = 12 hours to deliver the medication.

453. A patient's body surface area (BSA) is used to calculate medication dosages. If a patient weighs 70kg and is 1.75m tall, what is their BSA using the formula BSA = √(height(m)*weight(kg)/3600)?
a) 1.6 m²
b) 1.7 m²
c) 1.8 m²
d) 1.9 m²

Answer: b) 1.7 m². Explanation: Substituting the given values into the formula gives BSA = √(1.75*70/3600) ≈ 1.7 m².

454. A nurse needs to prepare a 15% saline solution for a patient. If she has a 100 ml of a 10% solution, how much of a 20% solution should she add to achieve this?
a) 50 ml
b) 75 ml
c) 100 ml
d) 125 ml

Answer: a) 50 ml. Explanation: If x is the volume of the 20% solution to add, we can set up the equation: 0.10100 + 0.20x = 0.15*(100 + x). Simplifying this gives x = 50 ml.

455. A doctor recommends a patient to consume 2000 calories per day. If the patient consumes 3 meals and 2 snacks per day, and wants each meal to supply twice as many calories as each snack, how many calories should each snack provide?
a) 200
b) 250
c) 300
d) 350

Answer: b) 250. Explanation: Let x be the number of calories in each snack. Then each meal provides 2x calories. So, 3 meals and 2 snacks provide 32x + 2x = 2000 calories, which solves to x = 250 calories.

456. A patient needs to have their blood pressure checked every 30 minutes for 4 hours. How many times will the nurse need to check the patient's blood pressure?
a) 7
b) 8
c) 9
d) 10

Answer: b) 8. Explanation: Over 4 hours, or 240 minutes, checking every 30 minutes will result in 240 / 30 = 8 checks.

457. A hospital room has an area of 300 square feet and needs to be disinfected. If a bottle of disinfectant covers 25 square feet, how many bottles are needed?
a) 10
b) 12
c) 14
d) 16

Answer: b) 12. Explanation: To find the number of bottles needed, divide the total area by the area covered by one bottle: 300 / 25 = 12 bottles.

458. If a nurse administers a medication at 8:00 am and the medication has a half-life of 6 hours, at what time will only 25% of the medication remain in the patient's system?
a) 2:00 pm
b) 8:00 pm
c) 2:00 am
d) 8:00 am the next day

Answer: a) 2:00 pm. Explanation: After one half-life (6 hours), 50% of the medication will remain. After another half-life (another 6 hours), half of this remaining amount will be left, so 50% of 50% is 25%. So, this would be 6 hours + 6 hours = 12 hours after the medication was administered, or 8:00 am + 12 hours = 8:00 pm.

459. A patient has been prescribed 2.5 liters of fluid intake per day. If the patient has already consumed 1.25 liters, what percentage of the prescribed fluid intake does the patient still need to consume?
a) 30%
b) 40%
c) 50%
d) 60%

Answer: c) 50%. Explanation: The patient still needs to consume 2.5 liters - 1.25 liters = 1.25 liters. This is 1.25/2.5 = 50% of the total prescribed fluid intake.

460. A doctor has advised a patient to reduce his daily sugar intake by 15%. If the patient usually consumes 40 grams of sugar daily, how many grams of sugar should he consume now?
a) 30 grams
b) 34 grams
c) 36 grams
d) 40 grams

Answer: b) 34 grams. Explanation: A 15% reduction in 40 grams is 40 - 0.15*40 = 34 grams.

461. A nurse needs to administer 300mg of a medication, but only has 100mg tablets available. How many tablets does she need to give?
a) 2
b) 3
c) 4
d) 5

Answer: b) 3. Explanation: To reach 300mg with 100mg tablets, the nurse needs 300/100 = 3 tablets.

462. A drug is administered every 4 hours. If the first dose was given at 8:00 AM, what time will the fifth dose be given?
a) 4:00 PM
b) 8:00 PM
c) 12:00 AM
d) 4:00 AM

Answer: a) 4:00 PM. Explanation: Each dose is given 4 hours apart, so the fifth dose will be given 4 * 4 = 16 hours after the first dose. 8:00 AM + 16 hours = 4:00 PM.

463. If a medication is supplied in 2 ml vials and a patient needs a 5 ml dose, how many vials are required?
a) 2
b) 3
c) 4
d) 5

Answer: b) 3. Explanation: To provide a 5 ml dose with 2 ml vials, you will need to use 5/2 = 2.5 vials. However, since you can't use half a vial, you'll need to round up to 3 vials.

464. The doctor advised a patient to consume 2500 kcal daily. If the patient's breakfast was 500 kcal, lunch was 700 kcal, and dinner was 900 kcal, how many kcal does the patient still need to consume to reach the daily goal?
a) 200 kcal
b) 300 kcal
c) 400 kcal
d) 500 kcal

Answer: c) 400 kcal. Explanation: The patient has already consumed 500 + 700 + 900 = 2100 kcal. Therefore, to reach the goal of 2500 kcal, the patient needs to consume 2500 - 2100 = 400 kcal more.

465. A nurse needs to dilute a 10 ml vial of medicine with a diluent to make a 20% solution. How much diluent does she need to add?
a) 10 ml
b) 20 ml
c) 30 ml
d) 40 ml

Answer: d) 40 ml. Explanation: In a 20% solution, the quantity of the substance (medicine) is 20% of the total quantity. Therefore, if 10 ml of medicine represents 20% of the solution, the total volume of the solution will be 10 ml / 0.2 = 50 ml. Since 10 ml is already medicine, the nurse needs to add 50 ml - 10 ml = 40 ml of diluent.

466. A patient has a fever of 103 degrees Fahrenheit. What is this in Celsius?
a) 38.3 degrees
b) 39.4 degrees
c) 39.5 degrees
d) 40.5 degrees

Answer: b) 39.4 degrees. Explanation: The formula to convert Fahrenheit to Celsius is (F - 32) * 5/9. Therefore, (103 - 32) * 5/9 = 39.4 degrees Celsius.

467. If a medication is to be given every 6 hours, how many times will it be given in a week?
a) 24 times
b) 28 times
c) 32 times
d) 42 times

Answer: d) 42 times. Explanation: There are 24 hours in a day, so medication given every 6 hours will be administered 24/6 = 4 times a day. Over a week (7 days), it will be given 4 * 7 = 28 times.

468. A clinic is open 5 days a week and sees 12 patients per day on average. How many patients does the clinic see in a month (assume 4 weeks in a month)?
a) 160
b) 200
c) 240
d) 280

Answer: c) 240. Explanation: The clinic is open for 5 days * 4 weeks = 20 days in a month. Seeing 12 patients per day, the clinic will see 20 * 12 = 240 patients in a month.

469. A patient is prescribed medication that needs to be taken twice a day for 10 days. If the medication comes in packs of 15, how many packs does the patient need to buy?
a) 1 pack
b) 2 packs
c) 3 packs
d) 4 packs

Answer: b) 2 packs. Explanation: The total amount of medication needed is 2 * 10 = 20. Since each pack contains 15 doses, the patient will need 20/15 = 1.33 packs, rounded up to 2 packs.

270. A patient needs to drink 3 liters of water a day. If they drink 8 glasses of water and each glass is 250 ml, did they reach the required amount?
a) Yes
b) No

Answer: b) No. Explanation: 8 glasses of water of 250 ml each gives 8 * 250 = 2000 ml or 2 liters. They are 1 liter short of the required amount.

471. A nurse needs to prepare a 250 ml saline solution with 5% salt. How many grams of salt does she need?
a) 5 grams
b) 12.5 grams
c) 25 grams
d) 50 grams

Answer: c) 25 grams. Explanation: 5% of 250 ml is 0.05 * 250 = 12.5 grams.

472. A patient has a fever of 102 degrees Fahrenheit. What is this in Celsius?
a) 36.7 degrees
b) 38.3 degrees
c) 38.9 degrees
d) 39.1 degrees

Answer: c) 38.9 degrees. Explanation: The formula to convert Fahrenheit to Celsius is (F - 32) * 5/9. Therefore, (102 - 32) * 5/9 = 38.9 degrees Celsius.

473. A doctor has prescribed a medication to be taken every 4 hours. How many doses will a patient take in one day?
a) 4 doses
b) 5 doses
c) 6 doses
d) 7 doses

Answer: c) 6 doses. Explanation: There are 24 hours in a day, so medication given every 4 hours will be administered 24/6 = 6 times a day.

474. A nurse needs to administer 1000mg of a medication, but only has 250mg tablets available. How many tablets does she need to give?
a) 2
b) 3
c) 4
d) 5

Answer: c) 4. Explanation: To reach 1000mg with 250mg tablets, the nurse needs 1000/250 = 4 tablets.

275. If a medication is to be given every 8 hours, how many times will it be given in a week?
a) 21 times
b) 24 times
c) 28 times
d) 42 times

Answer: a) 21 times. Explanation: There are 24 hours in a day, so medication given every 8 hours will be administered 24/8 = 3 times a day. Over a week (7 days), it will be given 3 * 7 = 21 times.

476. A patient needs to lose 15% of his body weight. If he currently weighs 200 pounds, how much will he weigh after he loses the weight?
a) 160 pounds
b) 170 pounds
c) 180 pounds
d) 190 pounds

Answer: b) 170 pounds. Explanation: 15% of 200 pounds is 200 * 0.15 = 30 pounds. After losing this weight, he will weigh 200 - 30 = 170 pounds.

477. A nurse needs to prepare 50 ml of a solution with 2% medication. How many ml of medication does she need to add to the solution?
a) 0.5 ml
b) 1 ml
c) 2 ml
d) 10 ml

Answer: b) 1 ml. Explanation: 2% of 50 ml is 0.02 * 50 = 1 ml.

478. A patient needs to take 500mg of a medication daily. If the medication comes in 100mg tablets, how many tablets should the patient take each day?
a) 3
b) 4
c) 5
d) 6

Answer: c) 5. Explanation: To reach 500mg with 100mg tablets, the patient needs 500/100 = 5 tablets.

479. A box of masks contains 50 masks. If a hospital ward uses 25 masks per day, how many days will one box last?
a) 1 day
b) 2 days
c) 3 days
d) 4 days

Answer: b) 2 days. Explanation: With a consumption of 25 masks per day, one box containing 50 masks will last for 50/25 = 2 days.

480. A prescription calls for 15mg/kg of a drug for a patient. If the patient weighs 68 kg, how many mg of the drug will be administered?
a) 510 mg
b) 1020 mg
c) 1530 mg
d) 2040 mg

Answer: c) 1530 mg. Explanation: Using the dosage formula (15mg/kg * patient's weight), we get 15*68 = 1020 mg.

481. If a nurse works a 12-hour shift and checks a patient's vitals every 4 hours, how many times will she check the patient's vitals during her shift?
a) 2
b) 3
c) 4
d) 5

Answer: c) 4. Explanation: During a 12-hour shift, a check every 4 hours would mean 12/4 = 3 checks. However, the first check is done at the beginning of the shift, so the total checks done are 3+1 = 4.

482. A doctor prescribes a medication to be given every 6 hours. How many times a day will this medication be given?
a) 3
b) 4
c) 5
d) 6

Answer: b) 4. Explanation: There are 24 hours in a day. If a medication is to be given every 6 hours, then it will be administered 24/6 = 4 times a day.

483. If a medication is given at a dosage of 250 mg every 8 hours, how much medication will be given in a 24-hour period?
a) 750 mg
b) 1000 mg
c) 1250 mg
d) 1500 mg

Answer: a) 750 mg. Explanation: In a 24-hour period, the medication will be given 24/8 = 3 times. Therefore, the total dosage is 3 * 250 mg = 750 mg.

484. A patient needs to receive 2000ml of IV fluid over a 12-hour period. If the drip rate of the IV is 20 drops/ml, how many drops per minute does the patient need?
a) 28 drops/minute
b) 33 drops/minute
c) 37 drops/minute
d) 42 drops/minute

Answer: a) 28 drops/minute. Explanation: There are 720 minutes in 12 hours, so the patient needs 2000ml/720minutes = 2.78 ml/minute. At a rate of 20 drops/ml, this is 2.78 ml/minute * 20 drops/ml = 55.56 drops/minute, rounded down to 28 drops/minute.

485. A nurse needs to administer 500 ml of fluid over 2 hours. If the drip factor of the IV tubing is 20 drops/ml, what should be the drip rate (drops/minute)?
a) 40 drops/minute
b) 50 drops/minute
c) 60 drops/minute
d) 70 drops/minute

Answer: b) 50 drops/minute. Explanation: The total amount of fluid (500ml) divided by the total time (120 minutes) is 4.17 ml/minute. Using the drip factor of 20 drops/ml, the drip rate should be 4.17 ml/minute * 20 drops/ml = 83.33 drops/minute, which rounded to the nearest whole number is 50 drops/minute.

486. If a patient drinks 8 ounces of water every hour for 10 hours, how many liters of water have they consumed? (1 ounce = 0.0295735 liters)
a) 0.7 liters
b) 2.4 liters
c) 3.5 liters
d) 4.7 liters

Answer: b) 2.4 liters. Explanation: The total amount of water consumed in liters is 8 ounces/hour * 10 hours * 0.0295735 liters/ounce = 2.36688 liters, rounded to 2.4 liters.

487. A doctor prescribes 300 mg of a medication to be taken twice daily. The medication is supplied in 150 mg tablets. How many tablets should the patient take in one day?
a) 2 tablets
b) 3 tablets
c) 4 tablets
d) 5 tablets

Answer: c) 4 tablets. Explanation: Each dose of 300 mg requires 2 tablets (300 mg/150 mg/tablet). Therefore, for two doses, the patient should take 2 tablets/dose * 2 doses/day = 4 tablets/day.

488. A carpenter has been hired to build a rectangular deck in a backyard. The deck is to be 15 feet long and 12 feet wide. What is the area of the deck?
a) 120 sq ft
b) 150 sq ft
c) 180 sq ft
d) 200 sq ft

Answer: c) 180 sq ft. Explanation: The area of a rectangle is calculated by multiplying the length by the width, so 15 ft * 12 ft = 180 sq ft.

489. A cylindrical canister has a diameter of 6 cm and a height of 10 cm. What is the volume of the canister? (Use the formula for the volume of a cylinder: V = πr^2h)
a) 120π cm^3
b) 180π cm^3
c) 280π cm^3
d) 360π cm^3

Answer: d) 360π cm^3. Explanation: The radius of the canister is half its diameter, or 3 cm. Thus, the volume is π*(3 cm)^2*10 cm = 90π cm^3.

490. A bag contains 5 red marbles, 4 green marbles, and 3 blue marbles. What is the probability of drawing a red marble from the bag?
a) 1/4
b) 1/3
c) 5/12
d) 1/2

Answer: c) 5/12. Explanation: There are a total of 12 marbles, and 5 of them are red. So, the probability of drawing a red marble is 5/12.

491. A box contains 6 red balls, 4 blue balls, and 5 green balls. If a ball is drawn at random from the box, what is the probability that it is not green?
a) 1/3
b) 1/2
c) 2/3
d) 5/6

Answer: c) 2/3. Explanation: There are 15 balls in total and 5 of them are green. So, there are 10 balls that are not green. The probability that a randomly drawn ball is not green is therefore 10/15 = 2/3.

492. A shop is selling apples at $1.50 per pound. How much would 7.5 pounds of apples cost?
a) $7.50
b) $11.25
c) $12.50
d) $15.00

Answer: b) $11.25. Explanation: At $1.50 per pound, 7.5 pounds of apples would cost $1.50 * 7.5 = $11.25.

493. A car travels at a constant speed of 60 miles per hour. How long would it take to travel 210 miles?
a) 2.5 hours
b) 3.5 hours
c) 4.5 hours
d) 5.5 hours

Answer: b) 3.5 hours. Explanation: At a speed of 60 miles per hour, it would take 210 miles / 60 miles per hour = 3.5 hours to travel 210 miles.

494. A recipe calls for 1 1/2 cups of flour for every 2/3 cup of sugar. How much flour is needed for 4 cups of sugar?
a) 2 1/4 cups
b) 4 1/2 cups
c) 6 cups
d) 9 cups

Answer: d) 9 cups. Explanation: The ratio of flour to sugar in the recipe is 1 1/2 : 2/3 = 9/2 : 2/3 = 27/2 : 2 = 13.5/1. So for 4 cups of sugar, you need 13.5 * 4 = 54/2 = 27 cups of flour.

495. The distance between Town A and Town B is 300 miles. A car is traveling from Town A to Town B at an average speed of 60 miles per hour. How long will it take to reach Town B?
a) 3 hours
b) 4 hours
c) 5 hours
d) 6 hours

Answer: c) 5 hours. Explanation: At a speed of 60 miles per hour, it would take 300 miles / 60 miles per hour = 5 hours to travel from Town A to Town B.

496. A restaurant sold 180 meals one evening. If 75% of these were vegetarian meals, how many vegetarian meals were sold?
a) 90 meals
b) 120 meals
c) 135 meals
d) 150 meals

Answer: c) 135 meals. Explanation: 75% of 180 is 0.75 * 180 = 135.

497. A spherical ball has a diameter of 6 cm. What is the volume of the ball? (Use the formula for the volume of a sphere: V = 4/3πr^3)
a) 36π cm^3
b) 72π cm^3
c) 144π cm^3
d) 288π cm^3

Answer: c) 144π cm^3. Explanation: The radius of the ball is half its diameter, or 3 cm. Thus, the volume is 4/3 * π * (3 cm)^3 = 4/3 * π * 27 cm^3 = 36π cm^3.

498. A patient needs to take 2 tablets every 4 hours. How many tablets will they need in one day?
a) 8 tablets
b) 12 tablets
c) 24 tablets
d) 48 tablets

Answer: c) 24 tablets. Explanation: A day has 24 hours. In each 4 hour period, the patient takes 2 tablets. Therefore, in 24 hours, the patient will need 24/4 * 2 = 24 tablets.

499. A car travels 150 miles on 10 gallons of gas. How many miles does the car get per gallon of gas?
a) 10 miles/gallon
b) 15 miles/gallon
c) 20 miles/gallon
d) 25 miles/gallon

Answer: b) 15 miles/gallon. Explanation: The car's fuel efficiency is calculated by dividing the total miles traveled by the total gallons of gas used. Therefore, 150 miles / 10 gallons = 15 miles/gallon.

500. A rectangular box measures 4 inches by 5 inches by 6 inches. What is the volume of the box?
a) 60 cubic inches
b) 90 cubic inches
c) 120 cubic inches
d) 150 cubic inches

Answer: c) 120 cubic inches. Explanation: The volume of a rectangular box is calculated by multiplying the length, width, and height. Therefore, 4 inches * 5 inches * 6 inches = 120 cubic inches.

501. A cake recipe requires 2/3 cup of sugar for every 1 1/2 cups of flour. How much sugar is needed if 4 1/2 cups of flour are used?
a) 1 cup
b) 2 cups
c) 3 cups
d) 4 cups

Answer: b) 2 cups. Explanation: The ratio of sugar to flour in the recipe is 2/3 : 1 1/2 = 4/6 : 9/6 = 2/3. Therefore, if 4 1/2 = 9/2 cups of flour are used, you would need 2/3 * 9/2 = 3 cups of sugar.

502. A store has a sale of 25% off all items. If an item originally costs $80, how much will it cost after the discount?
a) $20
b) $60
c) $70
d) $75

Answer: b) $60. Explanation: The discount is 25% of the original price, or 25/100 * $80 = $20. Therefore, the item will cost $80 - $20 = $60 after the discount.

503. A store buys a sweater for $40 and marks it up by 75%. How much is the sweater sold for?
a) $60
b) $70
c) $80
d) $100

Answer: b) $70. Explanation: The markup is 75% of the cost price, or 75/100 * $40 = $30. Therefore, the sweater is sold for $40 + $30 = $70.

504. A toy costs $15. After a 20% discount, what is the new price?
a) $10
b) $12
c) $13
d) $15

Answer: b) $12. Explanation: The discount is 20% of the original price, or 20/100 * $15 = $3. Therefore, the new price is $15 - $3 = $12.

505. A car travels 360 miles on 15 gallons of gas. How many miles does the car get per gallon of gas?
a) 20 miles/gallon
b) 24 miles/gallon
c) 25 miles/gallon
d) 30 miles/gallon

Answer: b) 24 miles/gallon. Explanation: The car's fuel efficiency is calculated by dividing the total miles traveled by the total gallons of gas used. Therefore, 360 miles / 15 gallons = 24 miles/gallon.

506. A rectangular box measures 8 inches by 3 inches by 2 inches. What is the volume of the box?
a) 16 cubic inches
b) 24 cubic inches
c) 48 cubic inches
d) 64 cubic inches

Answer: c) 48 cubic inches. Explanation: The volume of a rectangular box is calculated by multiplying the length, width, and height. Therefore, 8 inches * 3 inches * 2 inches = 48 cubic inches.

507. A bag contains 2 red, 3 blue, and 4 green marbles. What is the probability of drawing a blue marble?
a) 1/3
b) 1/2
c) 2/3
d) 3/4

Answer: a) 1/3. Explanation: The total number of marbles is 2 + 3 + 4 = 9. Therefore, the probability of drawing a blue marble is the number of blue marbles divided by the total number of marbles, or 3/9 = 1/3.

508. Which body system is responsible for coordinating and controlling the actions of all other body systems?
a) Digestive system
b) Respiratory system
c) Nervous system
d) Muscular system

Answer: c) Nervous system. Explanation: The nervous system is responsible for receiving information about the body and its environment, processing that information, and coordinating a response. It includes the brain, spinal cord, and nerves.

509. Which body system is primarily responsible for transporting oxygen, nutrients, hormones, and waste products throughout the body?
a) Cardiovascular system
b) Integumentary system
c) Endocrine system
d) Lymphatic system

Answer: a) Cardiovascular system. Explanation: The cardiovascular system, including the heart, blood, and blood vessels, is responsible for circulating blood throughout the body, which carries oxygen, nutrients, hormones, and waste products.

510. Which body system protects the body from environmental hazards and helps control body temperature?
a) Integumentary system
b) Respiratory system
c) Digestive system
d) Nervous system

Answer: a) Integumentary system. Explanation: The integumentary system, which includes the skin, hair, nails, and sweat glands, forms a protective barrier against environmental hazards and helps regulate body temperature through processes such as sweating.

511. What is the primary function of the respiratory system?
a) To coordinate body movement
b) To provide a physical barrier against environmental hazards
c) To filter out pathogens from the body
d) To bring oxygen into the body and remove carbon dioxide

Answer: d) To bring oxygen into the body and remove carbon dioxide. Explanation: The respiratory system, which includes the nose, mouth, throat, lungs, and the structures involved in the process of breathing, is primarily responsible for gas exchange: bringing in oxygen for the body to use and expelling waste carbon dioxide.

512. Which body system is primarily responsible for breaking down food into nutrients that the body can use?
a) Digestive system
b) Endocrine system
c) Muscular system
d) Immune system

Answer: a) Digestive system. Explanation: The digestive system, including the mouth, esophagus, stomach, small and large intestines, and associated glands, is primarily responsible for breaking down food into nutrients that can be absorbed and used by the body, and for eliminating undigested waste.

513. Which body system is responsible for producing hormones that regulate processes such as metabolism, growth, and mood?
a) Endocrine system
b) Nervous system
c) Lymphatic system
d) Muscular system

Answer: a) Endocrine system. Explanation: The endocrine system, which includes glands such as the pituitary, thyroid, adrenal, and pancreas, produces hormones that regulate many body processes, from metabolism and growth to mood and stress responses.

514. Which body system protects the body against disease and infection?
a) Immune system
b) Cardiovascular system
c) Muscular system
d) Skeletal system

Answer: a) Immune system. Explanation: The immune system, which includes the white blood cells, lymph nodes, and organs such as the spleen, is responsible for protecting the body against pathogens and other foreign substances, and for cleaning up dead cells and other debris within the body.

515. What is the primary function of the urinary system?
a) To coordinate the body's response to environmental stimuli
b) To protect the body against pathogens and other foreign substances
c) To filter the blood and remove waste products from the body
d) To provide a physical barrier against environmental hazards

Answer: c) To filter the blood and remove waste products from the body. Explanation: The urinary system, including the kidneys, ureters, bladder, and urethra, filters the blood to remove waste products, balances electrolytes, and regulates the amount of water in the body.

516. Which body system provides support and protection for the body, assists in movement, and produces blood cells?
a) Cardiovascular system
b) Skeletal system
c) Nervous system
d) Digestive system

Answer: b) Skeletal system. Explanation: The skeletal system, which includes bones, cartilage, ligaments, and tendons, provides support and protection for the body, assists in movement by providing a structure for muscle attachment, and produces blood cells in the bone marrow.

517. What is the primary function of the muscular system?
a) To provide a physical barrier against environmental hazards
b) To break down food into nutrients that the body can use
c) To coordinate the body's response to environmental stimuli
d) To enable movement and maintain posture

Answer: d) To enable movement and maintain posture. Explanation: The muscular system, which includes all the muscles in the body, is primarily responsible for enabling movement by contracting in response to neural stimulation, and for maintaining posture by creating a constant low-level contraction that holds the body in an upright position.

518. How does a malfunction in the endocrine system potentially affect other body systems?
a) It can prevent the transport of oxygen and nutrients.
b) It can impair the ability to break down and absorb nutrients.
c) It can disrupt the balance of hormones, affecting various bodily functions.
d) It doesn't affect other body systems.

Answer: c) It can disrupt the balance of hormones, affecting various bodily functions. Explanation: The endocrine system produces hormones, which regulate many body processes. A malfunction in this system can disrupt the balance of hormones, potentially affecting various body functions such as metabolism (digestive system), stress responses (nervous system), and more.

519. What could be a potential consequence of a problem with the urinary system?
a) Impaired digestion of food
b) Disrupted hormonal balance
c) Accumulation of waste products in the body
d) Decreased ability to fight infection

Answer: c) Accumulation of waste products in the body. Explanation: The urinary system filters the blood to remove waste products. If it's not functioning properly, these waste products can accumulate in the body, potentially leading to further health problems.

520. How could an issue with the immune system affect the overall health of the body?
a) It could disrupt the digestion and absorption of nutrients.
b) It could reduce the body's ability to fight off disease and infection.
c) It could prevent the proper circulation of blood.
d) It could lead to an inability to move or maintain posture.

Answer: b) It could reduce the body's ability to fight off disease and infection. Explanation: The immune system is responsible for protecting the body against pathogens and other foreign substances. If it's not functioning properly, the body may be more susceptible to disease and infection.

521. Which body system, if impaired, could directly impact the efficiency of gas exchange, potentially affecting all other body systems?
a) Digestive system
b) Respiratory system
c) Endocrine system
d) Immune system

Answer: b) Respiratory system. Explanation: The respiratory system is responsible for bringing in oxygen for the body to use and expelling waste carbon dioxide. If this system is impaired, it can reduce the efficiency of gas exchange, potentially affecting the function of all other body systems that rely on oxygen and removal of carbon dioxide.

522. How does a disease affecting the cardiovascular system potentially impact other body systems?
a) It could prevent the body from properly regulating temperature.
b) It could disrupt the balance of hormones in the body.
c) It could impair the transport of oxygen and nutrients to body tissues.
d) It could inhibit the body's ability to fight off disease and infection.

Answer: c) It could impair the transport of oxygen and nutrients to body tissues. Explanation: The cardiovascular system, including the heart, blood, and blood vessels, is responsible for circulating blood throughout the body. If this system is impaired, it could hinder the transport of oxygen and nutrients to body tissues, potentially affecting the function of all other body systems.

523. If the nervous system is compromised, which of the following is a potential outcome?
a) Inability to properly filter blood and excrete waste
b) Disruption in the absorption of nutrients from food
c) Difficulty in coordinating and controlling body functions
d) Impaired production of hormones regulating bodily functions

Answer: c) Difficulty in coordinating and controlling body functions. Explanation: The nervous system is responsible for receiving and processing information and coordinating responses. If it's compromised, this could cause difficulty in coordinating and controlling body functions.

524. A disruption in the digestive system could potentially lead to which of the following issues?
a) Impaired gas exchange
b) Reduced ability to fight off disease and infection
c) Inability to properly break down and absorb nutrients
d) Difficulty in coordinating and controlling body functions

Answer: c) Inability to properly break down and absorb nutrients. Explanation: The digestive system is responsible for breaking down food and absorbing nutrients. If there's a disruption in this system, it could potentially impair the body's ability to obtain the nutrients it needs for energy, growth, and repair.

525. How does a disease in the musculoskeletal system potentially affect overall health?
a) It could inhibit the body's ability to fight off disease and infection.
b) It could prevent the body from properly regulating temperature.
c) It could disrupt the balance of hormones in the body.
d) It can restrict movement and lead to general discomfort or pain.

Answer: d) It can restrict movement and lead to general discomfort or pain. Explanation: The musculoskeletal system supports movement and maintains posture. Any disease affecting this system can hinder mobility and cause pain or discomfort, which can affect overall quality of life.

526. What is the potential effect of a disease that affects the integumentary system (skin, hair, nails)?
a) It could disrupt the digestion and absorption of nutrients.
b) It could inhibit the body's ability to fight off disease and infection.
c) It could prevent the proper circulation of blood.
d) It could compromise the body's first line of defense against environmental factors.

Answer: d) It could compromise the body's first line of defense against environmental factors. Explanation: The integumentary system serves as the body's first line of defense against environmental factors. If this system is affected by disease, it could compromise this protective barrier and make the body more susceptible to infections and injuries.

527. What is the role of the hypothalamus in the human body?
a) It regulates the body's temperature.
b) It is responsible for muscular contraction.
c) It is the site of gas exchange in the lungs.
d) It aids in the digestion of food.

Answer: a) It regulates the body's temperature. Explanation: The hypothalamus is a small region of the brain. It's crucial for many important functions, including the regulation of body temperature, hunger, thirst, sleep, and emotional responses.

528. Which cell organelle is responsible for producing ATP, the cell's primary energy source?
a) The nucleus
b) The endoplasmic reticulum
c) The mitochondria
d) The golgi apparatus

Answer: c) The mitochondria. Explanation: The mitochondria, often referred to as the "powerhouse of the cell," are responsible for producing ATP (adenosine triphosphate), the cell's primary energy source.

529. What is the main function of the respiratory system?
a) To transport oxygen to the body's cells and remove carbon dioxide.
b) To control body movements and postures.
c) To produce hormones that regulate various bodily functions.
d) To protect the body from diseases and infections.

Answer: a) To transport oxygen to the body's cells and remove carbon dioxide. Explanation: The respiratory system is responsible for exchanging gases, primarily oxygen and carbon dioxide, between the body and the environment.

530. In the human body, where does blood cell production primarily occur?
a) The heart
b) The kidneys
c) The liver
d) The bone marrow

Answer: d) The bone marrow. Explanation: Blood cells are primarily produced in the bone marrow, the soft, spongy tissue found in the center of most bones.

531. What is the primary function of the pancreas?
a) It synthesizes proteins.
b) It produces hormones that regulate blood sugar levels.
c) It filters toxins from the blood.
d) It provides a defense against foreign invaders.

Answer: b) It produces hormones that regulate blood sugar levels. Explanation: The pancreas is responsible for producing hormones, including insulin and glucagon, that regulate blood sugar levels.

532. What role does the spinal cord play in the nervous system?
a) It serves as the primary storage site for memories.
b) It is the main site for gas exchange in the body.
c) It controls the body's voluntary movements.
d) It transmits information between the brain and the rest of the body.

Answer: d) It transmits information between the brain and the rest of the body. Explanation: The spinal cord is part of the central nervous system and acts as a conduit for signals between the brain and the rest of the body.

533. What is the main function of red blood cells (erythrocytes) in the human body?
a) They fight infections and diseases.
b) They carry oxygen from the lungs to the body's tissues.
c) They regulate blood clotting.
d) They remove waste products from the body.

Answer: b) They carry oxygen from the lungs to the body's tissues. Explanation: Red blood cells, or erythrocytes, are responsible for carrying oxygen from the lungs to the body's tissues and carbon dioxide from the tissues back to the lungs.

534. The synapse is a key structure in the nervous system. What occurs at this site?
a) Muscle contraction
b) Gas exchange
c) Signal transmission between neurons
d) Digestion of food

Answer: c) Signal transmission between neurons. Explanation: A synapse is a small gap at the end of a neuron that allows a signal to pass from one neuron to the next. This process of signal transmission is essential for communication within the nervous system.

535. Which type of tissue connects muscle to bone in the human body?
a) Adipose tissue
b) Tendons
c) Cartilage
d) Ligaments

Answer: b) Tendons. Explanation: Tendons are tough bands of fibrous connective tissue that connect muscle to bone and aid in movement of the joints.

536. What is the primary function of the circulatory system?
a) To control body temperature
b) To transport nutrients and oxygen to cells, and waste products away from cells.
c) To fight against disease and infection
d) To regulate sleep and other biological rhythms

Answer: b) To transport nutrients and oxygen to cells, and waste products away from cells. Explanation: The circulatory system, also known as the cardiovascular system, is responsible for transporting nutrients, oxygen, hormones, and other substances to cells and carrying away waste products like carbon dioxide.

537. What is the process by which a cell divides its DNA into two sets and splits to form two identical daughter cells?
a) Osmosis
b) Meiosis
c) Mitosis
d) Fermentation

Answer: c) Mitosis. Explanation: Mitosis is the process by which a cell duplicates its DNA and divides into two genetically identical daughter cells. This process is essential for growth and repair in organisms.

538. What type of biological molecule are enzymes?
a) Carbohydrates
b) Lipids
c) Proteins
d) Nucleic acids

Answer: c) Proteins. Explanation: Enzymes are proteins that act as biological catalysts, speeding up chemical reactions in the body without being consumed in the process.

539. In genetics, what does the term "homozygous" mean?
a) The two alleles for a trait are different.
b) The two alleles for a trait are the same.
c) The alleles are located on the X and Y chromosomes.
d) The alleles are responsible for multiple traits.

Answer: b) The two alleles for a trait are the same. Explanation: In genetics, an individual is homozygous for a trait if they carry two copies of the same allele.

540. What is the primary function of the ribosomes in a cell?
a) To produce energy.
b) To synthesize proteins.
c) To transport materials within the cell.
d) To protect the cell from its environment.

Answer: b) To synthesize proteins. Explanation: Ribosomes are cell structures that make proteins from amino acids, a process known as protein synthesis.

541. Which term describes the movement of water from an area of lower solute concentration to an area of higher solute concentration?
a) Osmosis
b) Diffusion
c) Active transport
d) Endocytosis

Answer: a) Osmosis. Explanation: Osmosis is the process in which water molecules move from an area of lower solute concentration to an area of higher solute concentration, typically across a semipermeable membrane.

542. What is the role of the chloroplasts in a plant cell?
a) They break down glucose to produce energy.
b) They synthesize proteins.
c) They carry out photosynthesis.
d) They package and distribute proteins.

Answer: c) They carry out photosynthesis. Explanation: Chloroplasts are organelles found in plant cells that capture light energy and convert it into chemical energy through the process of photosynthesis.

543. Which of the following is a key difference between DNA and RNA?
a) DNA is double-stranded, while RNA is single-stranded.
b) DNA contains the sugar ribose, while RNA contains the sugar deoxyribose.
c) DNA is found only in the nucleus, while RNA is found only in the cytoplasm.
d) DNA carries amino acids, while RNA does not.

Answer: a) DNA is double-stranded, while RNA is single-stranded. Explanation: One of the key differences between DNA and RNA is their structure: DNA is typically double-stranded, while RNA is single-stranded.

544. What term describes an organism's observable traits or characteristics?
a) Genotype
b) Phenotype
c) Haploid
d) Homozygous

Answer: b) Phenotype. Explanation: An organism's phenotype refers to its observable physical properties or traits, such as its appearance, development, and behavior. These traits are determined by the organism's genetic makeup and environmental influences.

545. What is the process by which plants convert light energy into chemical energy in the form of glucose or other sugars?
a) Respiration
b) Photosynthesis
c) Fermentation
d) Glycolysis

Answer: b) Photosynthesis. Explanation: Photosynthesis is the process by which green plants, algae, and some bacteria convert light energy, usually from the Sun, into chemical energy in the form of glucose or other sugars.

546. In biology, what is a genome?
a) The complete set of genes or genetic material present in a cell or organism.
b) The study of heredity and the variation of inherited characteristics.
c) The structure within a cell that bears the genetic material as a threadlike linear strand of DNA bonded with various proteins.
d) The cellular process of producing proteins by decoding the information in messenger RNA.

Answer: a) The complete set of genes or genetic material present in a cell or organism. Explanation: A genome refers to all of the genes or genetic material in an organism or a cell. It includes both the genes (the coding regions) and the noncoding DNA, as well as the genetic material of the mitochondria and/or chloroplasts.

547. Which component of a cell is responsible for controlling what enters and leaves the cell?
a) Nucleus
b) Mitochondria
c) Cell membrane
d) Ribosomes

Answer: c) Cell membrane. Explanation: The cell membrane, also known as the plasma membrane, controls the movement of substances in and out of cells and protects the cell from its environment.

548. Which structure is often referred to as the "powerhouse" of the cell due to its role in energy production?
a) Endoplasmic reticulum
b) Ribosomes
c) Mitochondria
d) Nucleus

Answer: c) Mitochondria. Explanation: The mitochondria are the sites of cellular respiration and energy production in the cell, earning them the nickname "powerhouse of the cell."

549. What is the primary function of the nucleus in a cell?
a) Protein synthesis
b) Digestion of cellular waste
c) Regulation of cell metabolism and growth
d) Energy production

Answer: c) Regulation of cell metabolism and growth. Explanation: The nucleus contains the cell's genetic material and controls the cell's growth and reproduction.

550. What is the function of ribosomes in a cell?
a) To provide energy for the cell
b) To control the cell's activities
c) To produce proteins
d) To maintain cell shape

Answer: c) To produce proteins. Explanation: Ribosomes are the site of protein synthesis in the cell, creating proteins according to the instructions from DNA.

551. Which of the following cell structures is responsible for packaging and sorting proteins for delivery to their final destinations?
a) Endoplasmic reticulum
b) Ribosomes
c) Golgi apparatus
d) Mitochondria

Answer: c) Golgi apparatus. Explanation: The Golgi apparatus modifies, sorts, and packages proteins for transport to their final destinations.

552. The cell wall is a feature present in:
a) Animal cells only
b) Plant cells only
c) Both animal and plant cells
d) Neither animal nor plant cells

Answer: b) Plant cells only. Explanation: The cell wall is a rigid layer that provides support and protection to plant cells. Animal cells do not have a cell wall.

553. What is the primary role of the endoplasmic reticulum in a cell?
a) It breaks down toxic substances and digests fats.
b) It is where photosynthesis occurs.
c) It synthesizes and transports proteins and lipids.
d) It assists in the division of cells.

Answer: c) It synthesizes and transports proteins and lipids. Explanation: The endoplasmic reticulum is involved in the synthesis of proteins and lipids, which are vital for the cell's functioning.

554. The mitochondria and the chloroplasts are similar in that they both:
a) Are only found in plant cells.
b) Have a double membrane.
c) Are the site of protein synthesis.
d) Contain the cell's genetic material.

Answer: b) Have a double membrane. Explanation: Both mitochondria and chloroplasts are bound by a double membrane and have their own DNA.

556. What is the function of lysosomes in a cell?
a) DNA replication
b) Synthesis of proteins
c) Digestion of macromolecules
d) Production of energy

Answer: c) Digestion of macromolecules. Explanation: Lysosomes contain enzymes that break down waste materials and cellular debris.

557. Which part of a cell serves as the site for lipid synthesis and detoxification of harmful metabolic byproducts?
a) Golgi apparatus
b) Smooth Endoplasmic Reticulum
c) Rough Endoplasmic Reticulum
d) Nucleus

Answer: b) Smooth Endoplasmic Reticulum. Explanation: The smooth endoplasmic reticulum is responsible for lipid synthesis and detoxification of metabolic byproducts.

558. What is the term for the process by which DNA is used as a template to create messenger RNA (mRNA)?
a) Transcription
b) Translation
c) Replication
d) Mutation

Answer: a) Transcription. Explanation: Transcription is the process of creating an mRNA strand from a DNA template, which is a critical step in protein synthesis.

559. Personalized medicine often relies on understanding an individual's _____ to provide targeted treatment.
a) Genome
b) Proteome
c) Metabolome
d) All of the above

Answer: d) All of the above. Explanation: Personalized medicine considers a person's unique genetic makeup (genome), protein products (proteome), and metabolic profile (metabolome) to provide treatment most likely to be effective for them.

560. What is the term for a change in the DNA sequence that can lead to a different protein being produced?
a) Translation
b) Transcription
c) Replication
d) Mutation

Answer: d) Mutation. Explanation: A mutation is a change in the DNA sequence that can potentially lead to a different protein being produced, which can influence an organism's traits and potentially cause disease.

561. The sequencing of the human genome has primarily impacted medicine by:
a) Making it possible to predict all diseases a person will get
b) Providing the blueprint for all human proteins
c) Identifying the genes responsible for hair color
d) Allowing doctors to create personalized exercise plans

Answer: b) Providing the blueprint for all human proteins. Explanation: The sequencing of the human genome has provided a blueprint for human proteins, allowing scientists to identify genes associated with diseases and understand their functions.

562. Which technique is used in modern medicine to replace a faulty gene with a functioning one in patients?
a) Gene therapy
b) Cloning
c) PCR
d) Microscopy

Answer: a) Gene therapy. Explanation: Gene therapy is a technique that uses genes to treat or prevent disease. In the future, this technique may allow doctors to treat a disorder by inserting a gene into a patient's cells instead of using drugs or surgery.

563. What role does understanding protein structure play in drug design?
a) It helps to identify potential drug targets
b) It allows for the creation of drugs that can specifically bind to and alter the function of target proteins
c) It helps to predict the effects of mutations on protein function
d) All of the above

Answer: d) All of the above. Explanation: Understanding protein structure plays a critical role in drug design. It helps to identify potential drug targets, allows for the creation of drugs that specifically interact with those targets, and helps to predict the effects of mutations on protein function.

564. What does the term 'pharmacogenomics' refer to?
a) The study of how genes affect a person's response to drugs
b) The study of the structure of drug molecules
c) The study of the side effects of drugs
d) The study of drug addiction

Answer: a) The study of how genes affect a person's response to drugs. Explanation: Pharmacogenomics is the study of how a person's genes influence their body's response to drugs. It can help to predict who will benefit from a medication, who will not respond at all, and who will experience negative side effects.

565. How do genetic tests contribute to modern medicine?
a) They can confirm or rule out a suspected genetic condition
b) They can predict the likelihood of developing a genetic disorder
c) They can help determine a person's chance of passing on a genetic disorder to their children
d) All of the above

Answer: d) All of the above. Explanation: Genetic tests have a broad range of uses in modern medicine, including confirming or ruling out suspected genetic conditions, predicting the likelihood of developing certain diseases, and helping determine a person's chance of passing on a genetic disorder to their children.

566. What technology allows scientists to easily and selectively edit genes within organisms?
a) PCR
b) CRISPR
c) Gel electrophoresis
d) DNA sequencing

Answer: b) CRISPR. Explanation: CRISPR (Clustered Regularly Interspaced Short Palindromic Repeats) is a revolutionary technology that allows scientists to easily and selectively edit the genes of organisms, including humans.

567. Which of the following is not a product of transcription?
a) mRNA
b) tRNA
c) rRNA
d) DNA

Answer: d) DNA. Explanation: Transcription produces three types of RNA: messenger RNA (mRNA), transfer RNA (tRNA), and ribosomal RNA (rRNA). DNA, on the other hand, is the template used in transcription, not a product of it.

568. How many protons are in the nucleus of an atom of carbon (atomic number 6)?
a) 6
b) 12
c) 18
d) 24

Answer: a) 6. Explanation: The atomic number of an element corresponds to the number of protons in the nucleus of an atom of that element. Therefore, an atom of carbon, which has an atomic number of 6, has 6 protons.

569. The atomic weight of magnesium (Mg) is 24 and its atomic number is 12. How many neutrons does magnesium have?
a) 12
b) 24
c) 36
d) 48

Answer: a) 12. Explanation: The atomic weight is the sum of the number of protons and neutrons. Since the atomic number is the number of protons and equals 12 for magnesium, the number of neutrons is also 12 (24-12).

570. Which type of chemical bond results from the transfer of electrons from one atom to another?
a) Covalent bond
b) Hydrogen bond
c) Ionic bond
d) Metallic bond

Answer: c) Ionic bond. Explanation: An ionic bond is a type of chemical bond that involves a metal and a nonmetal ion (or polyatomic ions such as ammonium) through electrostatic attraction. It results from the transfer of electrons from one atom to another, creating ions that are attracted to each other.

571. What happens during a neutralization reaction?
a) An acid reacts with a base to produce salt and water
b) An acid reacts with a metal to produce salt and hydrogen
c) A base reacts with a metal to produce salt and water
d) An acid and a base react to produce only water

Answer: a) An acid reacts with a base to produce salt and water. Explanation: A neutralization reaction occurs when an acid reacts with a base and produces a salt and water.

572. What is the pH of a neutral solution at 25°C?
a) 0
b) 7
c) 14
d) 100

Answer: b) 7. Explanation: At 25°C, a neutral solution has a pH of 7. pH values lower than 7 indicate an acidic solution, while pH values higher than 7 indicate a basic solution.

573. Which of the following is not a characteristic of a base?
a) Tastes bitter
b) Feels slippery
c) Turns litmus paper red
d) Reacts with acids to produce salts

Answer: c) Turns litmus paper red. Explanation: Bases have a bitter taste, feel slippery, and turn litmus paper blue. It is acids that turn litmus paper red.

574. What is the molar mass of water (H2O)?
a) 18 g/mol
b) 20 g/mol
c) 22 g/mol
d) 24 g/mol

Answer: a) 18 g/mol. Explanation: The molar mass of water is calculated by adding the molar mass of two hydrogen atoms (2*1 g/mol) to the molar mass of one oxygen atom (16 g/mol). This gives a total of 18 g/mol.

575. The atomic number of sodium is 11. How many electrons are in a neutral atom of sodium?
a) 11
b) 22
c) 33
d) 44

Answer: a) 11. Explanation: A neutral atom has an equal number of protons and electrons. Since the atomic number of sodium, which represents the number of protons, is 11, a neutral atom of sodium also has

576. What is the number of atoms in one mole of a substance?
a) 6.022 x 10^23 atoms
b) 1.66 x 10^-24 atoms
c) 3.14 x 10^7 atoms
d) 2.82 x 10^26 atoms

Answer: a) 6.022 x 10^23 atoms. Explanation: Avogadro's number, 6.022 x 10^23, is the number of atoms or molecules in one mole of any substance.

577. A chemist has 22.4 L of a gas at STP (standard temperature and pressure). How many moles of gas does she have?
a) 1 mole
b) 22.4 moles
c) 44.8 moles
d) 89.6 moles

Answer: a) 1 mole. Explanation: At STP, one mole of any gas occupies a volume of 22.4 L.

578. Which of the following statements is a law of conservation of mass?
a) Matter cannot be created or destroyed in a chemical reaction
b) Energy cannot be created or destroyed, but it can be transformed from one form to another
c) In a chemical reaction, the sum of the masses of the reactants equals the sum of the masses of the products
d) Both a) and c)

Answer: d) Both a) and c). Explanation: The law of conservation of mass states that matter cannot be created or destroyed in a chemical reaction (a), and in a chemical reaction, the sum of the masses of the reactants equals the sum of the masses of the products (c).

579. What is the name of a substance that speeds up a chemical reaction without being consumed by the reaction?
a) Reactant
b) Product
c) Catalyst
d) Solvent

Answer: c) Catalyst. Explanation: A catalyst is a substance that speeds up a chemical reaction by lowering the activation energy, but is not consumed by the reaction.

580. What happens to the particles of a gas as its temperature increases?
a) They move more slowly
b) They move more quickly
c) They become larger
d) They become smaller

Answer: b) They move more quickly. Explanation: As the temperature of a gas increases, the kinetic energy of the gas particles increases, causing them to move more quickly.

581. What is the term for the amount of energy required to change a substance from a liquid to a gas at its boiling point?
a) Enthalpy of vaporization
b) Enthalpy of fusion
c) Enthalpy of sublimation
d) Enthalpy of combustion

Answer: a) Enthalpy of vaporization. Explanation: The enthalpy of vaporization is the amount of energy required to change a substance from a liquid to a gas at its boiling point.

582. Which state of matter has a definite volume but no definite shape?
a) Solid
b) Liquid
c) Gas
d) Plasma

Answer: b) Liquid. Explanation: A liquid has a definite volume but no definite shape. It takes the shape of its container.

583. What is the term for the temperature and pressure conditions at which the solid, liquid, and gaseous phases of a substance coexist at equilibrium?
a) Triple point
b) Critical point
c) Boiling point
d) Freezing point

Answer: a) Triple point. Explanation: The triple point of a substance is the temperature and pressure at which the three phases (gas, liquid, and solid) of that substance coexist in thermodynamic equilibrium.

584. Which part of an atom carries a positive charge?
a) Proton
b) Neutron
c) Electron
d) Nucleus

Answer: a) Proton. Explanation: In an atom, protons carry a positive charge. They are located in the nucleus along with neutrons, which carry no charge. Electrons, which carry a negative charge, move in the space around the nucleus.

585. What does the atomic number of an element represent?
a) The number of protons
b) The number of neutrons
c) The number of electrons
d) The total number of protons and neutrons

Answer: a) The number of protons. Explanation: The atomic number of an element is equal to the number of protons in the nucleus of its atom.

586. Isotopes of the same element have different numbers of what?
a) Protons
b) Neutrons
c) Electrons
d) Nuclei

Answer: b) Neutrons. Explanation: Isotopes of the same element have the same number of protons (and therefore the same atomic number) but different numbers of neutrons. This means they have different atomic masses.

587. Which type of atomic particle contributes to the mass of the atom but does not affect its chemical properties?
a) Protons
b) Neutrons
c) Electrons
d) Both a) and b)

Answer: b) Neutrons. Explanation: The number of neutrons in an atom does not affect its chemical properties, which are determined by the number of protons (atomic number) and electrons. Neutrons do, however, contribute to the mass of the atom.

585. Why is an understanding of atomic structure important in the field of medicine?
a) It's not really relevant
b) It helps in the development of new drugs and treatments
c) It's important for understanding how radiation affects the body
d) Both b) and c)

Answer: d) Both b) and c). Explanation: An understanding of atomic structure is crucial in medicine for developing new drugs and treatments, as well as for understanding how radiation affects the body.

586. Which type of radiation is made up of two protons and two neutrons?
a) Alpha particles
b) Beta particles
c) Gamma rays
d) X-rays

Answer: a) Alpha particles. Explanation: Alpha particles consist of two protons and two neutrons. They are relatively large and are therefore the least penetrating form of radiation, but they can cause damage if they are ingested or inhaled.

587. Which of the following is a common use of radioactive isotopes in medicine?
a) In chemotherapy to target and kill cancer cells
b) As tracers to study the function of organs or tissues
c) In radiation therapy to kill tumors
d) All of the above

Answer: d) All of the above. Explanation: Radioactive isotopes, also known as radioisotopes, are used in medicine for various purposes, including in chemotherapy to target and kill cancer cells, as tracers to study the function of organs or tissues, and in radiation therapy to kill tumors.

588. Which of the following accurately describes the location of electrons within an atom?
a) They orbit the nucleus in fixed paths called orbits
b) They exist in a cloud-like formation around the nucleus known as the electron cloud
c) They reside within the nucleus along with the protons and neutrons
d) They freely float throughout the atom

Answer: b) They exist in a cloud-like formation around the nucleus known as the electron cloud. Explanation: In an atom, electrons are found in an area around the nucleus known as the electron cloud. They are not found in fixed paths or orbits.

589. The atomic mass of an atom is determined by the sum of which atomic particles?
a) Protons and Electrons
b) Neutrons and Electrons
c) Protons and Neutrons
d) Protons, Neutrons, and Electrons

Answer: c) Protons and Neutrons. Explanation: The atomic mass is calculated by adding the number of protons and neutrons in an atom. The mass of electrons is very small and does not significantly contribute to the overall atomic mass.

590. Why is the concept of half-life important in medicine, particularly in radiology?
a) It indicates how quickly a radioactive substance will decay
b) It determines the duration of effectiveness for a drug
c) It explains how quickly a patient will recover from surgery
d) It's not relevant in medicine

Answer: a) It indicates how quickly a radioactive substance will decay. Explanation: Half-life is a crucial concept in radiology and nuclear medicine as it indicates the time required for half of the radioactive atoms in a sample to decay. This information helps in determining the dosage and timing for treatments involving radioactive substances.

591. What is the significance of valence electrons in the formation of chemical bonds?
a) They participate in bond formation as they are in the atom's outermost shell
b) They have no role in bond formation
c) They prevent bond formation
d) They only participate in ionic bond formation

Answer: a) They participate in bond formation as they are in the atom's outermost shell. Explanation: Valence electrons, which are the electrons in the outermost shell of an atom, are involved in the formation of chemical bonds with other atoms.

592. What role does the understanding of atomic structure and radioactivity play in cancer treatment?
a) It's essential for developing radiation therapies that target cancer cells
b) It helps in designing drugs that can penetrate the nuclear envelope of cancer cells
c) It has no role in cancer treatment
d) It's necessary for predicting the patient's response to treatment

Answer: a) It's essential for developing radiation therapies that target cancer cells. Explanation: The understanding of atomic structure and radioactivity is crucial for developing radiation therapies that can effectively target and kill cancer cells while minimizing damage to healthy cells.

593. How is the knowledge of ionizing radiation important in healthcare?
a) It aids in understanding the effects and risks of radiation therapy
b) It is crucial for the operation and use of medical imaging devices like X-rays and CT scans
c) It helps to understand the sterilization of medical equipment
d) All of the above

Answer: d) All of the above. Explanation: Knowledge of ionizing radiation, which refers to radiation with enough energy to remove tightly bound electrons from atoms, thus creating ions, is important in healthcare for various reasons. It aids in understanding the effects and risks of radiation therapy, is crucial for the operation and use of medical imaging devices like X-rays and CT scans, and also helps to understand the sterilization of medical equipment.

594. What type of bonding is primarily responsible for the unique three-dimensional shape of proteins in the body?
a) Ionic bonding
b) Covalent bonding
c) Hydrogen bonding
d) Metallic bonding

Answer: c) Hydrogen bonding. Explanation: While proteins are primarily formed through covalent bonds (specifically peptide bonds), the unique three-dimensional structure of proteins is largely due to hydrogen bonding. These bonds influence the folding and shape of the protein, which in turn affects the protein's function in the body.

595. Which subatomic particles contribute to an atom's mass number?
a) Protons and Electrons
b) Neutrons and Electrons
c) Protons and Neutrons
d) Electrons only

Answer: c) Protons and Neutrons. Explanation: An atom's mass number is the total number of protons and neutrons in its nucleus. Electrons, while part of the atom's structure, are so small their contribution to the overall mass is negligible.

596. In radiology, what does the term "contrast" refer to?
a) The color scheme used in the images
b) The difference in densities between two tissues, making them distinguishable
c) The size of the structures in the image
d) The speed at which the image is produced

Answer: b) The difference in densities between two tissues, making them distinguishable. Explanation: In radiology, contrast refers to the difference in densities between two tissues, which allows them to be distinguished from each other on an imaging study. This concept is crucial to the field of medical imaging, which relies on differences in atomic structure and density to create detailed images of the body's interior.

597. What is the relevance of the Pauli Exclusion Principle in medical diagnostics?
a) It helps in understanding the working of MRI scanners
b) It explains the basis of X-ray imaging
c) It is crucial for the development of new medications
d) It has no relevance in medical diagnostics

Answer: a) It helps in understanding the working of MRI scanners. Explanation: The Pauli Exclusion Principle states that no two electrons in an atom can have the same four quantum numbers. This principle is vital in understanding the behavior of atomic particles in the presence of a magnetic field, which is the fundamental principle behind Magnetic Resonance Imaging (MRI) scanners.

598. In the human body, why is the understanding of the properties of water and its importance as a solvent significant?
a) It helps to understand the dissolution and transport of nutrients and wastes
b) It is vital for understanding the processes of digestion and absorption
c) It is important for maintaining the body's temperature
d) All of the above

Answer: d) All of the above. Explanation: Water's properties as a solvent, its high specific heat, and its role in digestion and absorption make it essential for various physiological processes in the body, including the transport of nutrients and wastes, maintaining body temperature, and aiding in digestion and absorption.

599. What is the role of diffusion in the human body?
a) It is a key mechanism for the transport of substances within cells
b) It assists in the generation of electrical signals in the nervous system
c) It helps in the maintenance of body temperature
d) It aids in the clotting of blood

Answer: a) It is a key mechanism for the transport of substances within cells. Explanation: Diffusion is the passive movement of molecules from an area of higher concentration to an area of lower concentration. In the body, it plays a significant role in the transport of substances within cells and across cell membranes.

600. The process by which our body breaks down food into smaller particles is an example of what type of change?
a) Physical change
b) Chemical change
c) Both physical and chemical change
d) Neither physical nor chemical change

Answer: c) Both physical and chemical change. Explanation: The digestion process involves both physical changes (such as chewing and churning in the stomach) and chemical changes (such as enzymatic breakdown of food particles).

601. How does the concept of osmosis apply to the human body?
a) It assists in the absorption of nutrients in the intestines
b) It helps in the regulation of body temperature
c) It aids in the conduction of nerve impulses
d) It assists in the clotting of blood

Answer: a) It assists in the absorption of nutrients in the intestines. Explanation: Osmosis, the passive movement of water across a semi-permeable membrane from an area of lower solute concentration to an area of higher solute concentration, is crucial in the body for various processes, including the absorption of water and nutrients in the intestines.

602. Why is the understanding of pH and acid-base balance critical in healthcare?
a) It's important for understanding the functionality of the digestive system
b) It's crucial for maintaining homeostasis and normal bodily functions
c) It plays a vital role in the conduction of nerve impulses
d) It has no significance in healthcare

Answer: b) It's crucial for maintaining homeostasis and normal bodily functions. Explanation: Acid-base balance, often measured by pH, is crucial in maintaining homeostasis in the body. A slight change in pH can significantly affect many physiological processes and the functioning of enzymes.

603. What is the relevance of understanding the states of matter in physiology?
a) It helps understand the different forms in which drugs can be administered
b) It's not relevant in physiology
c) It aids in understanding the clotting of blood
d) It assists in understanding the conduction of nerve impulses

Answer: a) It helps understand the different forms in which drugs can be administered. Explanation: Understanding the states of matter - solid, liquid, and gas - is important in physiology, particularly when it comes to the administration of drugs. For instance, drugs can be administered in various forms like tablets (solid), injections (liquid), and inhalers (gas).

604. How do the properties of gases apply to the functioning of the respiratory system?
a) They assist in the process of breathing, which relies on changes in pressure
b) They help in the conduction of nerve impulses
c) They aid in the maintenance of body temperature
d) They are not relevant to the functioning of the respiratory system

Answer: a) They assist in the process of breathing, which relies on changes in pressure. Explanation: The properties of gases, particularly their ability to expand and contract with changes in pressure, play a critical role in the process of breathing. The respiratory system relies on changes in pressure to inhale (draw in) and exhale (push out) air.

605. How does the concept of specific heat capacity apply to the human body?
a) It aids in the absorption of nutrients in the intestines
b) It helps in the maintenance of body temperature
c) It assists in the conduction of nerve impulses
d) It has no significance in the human body

Answer: b) It helps in the maintenance of body temperature. Explanation: Specific heat capacity refers to the amount of heat required to raise the temperature of a substance. Water, which makes up a large portion of the human body, has a high specific heat capacity, helping the body resist changes in temperature.

606. Why is understanding of the law of conservation of energy important in understanding human metabolism?
a) It explains how energy cannot be created or destroyed, but only transformed, such as in the conversion of food into energy
b) It aids in the absorption of nutrients in the intestines
c) It assists in the clotting of blood
d) It has no relevance in understanding human metabolism

Answer: a) It explains how energy cannot be created or destroyed, but only transformed, such as in the conversion of food into energy. Explanation: The law of conservation of energy, stating that energy cannot be created or destroyed but only transformed, is central to understanding how the body converts food into energy (in the form of ATP) through metabolic processes.

607. What type of chemical reaction is primarily responsible for the release of energy in the body?
a) Synthesis reaction
b) Decomposition reaction
c) Acid-base reaction
d) Redox reaction

Answer: d) Redox reaction. Explanation: Redox reactions, or oxidation-reduction reactions, involve the transfer of electrons and are responsible for the body's primary method of energy production, including the process of cellular respiration where glucose is oxidized to produce ATP.

608. How does the understanding of enzymatic reactions contribute to the development of drugs?
a) It helps design drugs that can inhibit or enhance enzymatic reactions
b) It aids in the development of drug delivery methods
c) It assists in predicting the side effects of drugs
d) It has no significance in drug development

Answer: a) It helps design drugs that can inhibit or enhance enzymatic reactions. Explanation: Understanding how enzymes function can aid in the design of drugs that can inhibit or enhance certain enzymatic reactions, thereby influencing the course of certain physiological processes or diseases.

609. Why are buffers important in maintaining the body's pH balance?
a) They assist in the absorption of nutrients
b) They help in the regulation of body temperature
c) They resist changes in pH by neutralizing added acids or bases
d) They are not significant in maintaining the body's pH balance

Answer: c) They resist changes in pH by neutralizing added acids or bases. Explanation: Buffers play a crucial role in maintaining the body's pH balance. They resist drastic changes in pH by neutralizing added acids or bases.

610. Why is the understanding of the process of hydrolysis important in the context of digestion?
a) It aids in the absorption of nutrients
b) It describes the breaking down of large molecules into smaller ones with the addition of water
c) It assists in maintaining body temperature
d) It has no relevance in the process of digestion

Answer: b) It describes the breaking down of large molecules into smaller ones with the addition of water. Explanation: Hydrolysis is a chemical reaction that breaks down large molecules into smaller ones with the addition of water. This process is central to digestion, as it allows the body to break down complex food substances into simpler, absorbable nutrients.

611. What role do oxidation-reduction reactions play in human physiology?
a) They help maintain body temperature
b) They play a crucial role in energy production through processes like cellular respiration
c) They assist in the absorption of nutrients
d) They aid in the clotting of blood

Answer: b) They play a crucial role in energy production through processes like cellular respiration. Explanation: Oxidation-reduction (redox) reactions are fundamental to several biochemical processes, including energy production through cellular respiration. In these reactions, electrons are transferred from one molecule (the reducing agent) to another (the oxidizing agent), often releasing energy in the process.

612. How does an understanding of chemical reactions contribute to the field of pharmacology?
a) It aids in the development of new drug delivery methods
b) It assists in understanding how drugs interact with the body at a molecular level
c) It helps in predicting the side effects of drugs
d) It has no relevance in pharmacology

Answer: b) It assists in understanding how drugs interact with the body at a molecular level. Explanation: Understanding chemical reactions is crucial in pharmacology as it helps in understanding how drugs interact with the body at a molecular level, how they are metabolized, and how they exert their therapeutic effects.

613. What is the role of dehydration synthesis in the human body?
a) It aids in the maintenance of body temperature
b) It helps in the absorption of nutrients
c) It is responsible for the formation of large molecules by removing water
d) It has no significance in the human body

Answer: c) It is responsible for the formation of large molecules by removing water. Explanation: Dehydration synthesis is a chemical reaction that involves the formation of a large molecule from smaller subunits, with the removal of a water molecule. This process is involved in the synthesis of several types of macromolecules in the body, including proteins and nucleic acids.

614. Why is understanding chemical equilibrium important in the context of human physiology?
a) It aids in understanding how the body maintains homeostasis
b) It helps in the regulation of body temperature
c) It assists in the absorption of nutrients
d) It has no relevance in human physiology

Answer: a) It aids in understanding how the body maintains homeostasis. Explanation: Chemical equilibrium is a state in a chemical reaction where the concentration of reactants and products remains constant over time. Understanding this concept is crucial in physiology as many biological processes are regulated to maintain equilibrium, thus helping the body maintain homeostasis.

615. What role does the principle of Le Chatelier's play in understanding human physiology?
a) It aids in understanding how the body responds to changes in order to maintain homeostasis
b) It assists in the absorption of nutrients
c) It helps in the regulation of body temperature
d) It has no relevance in human physiology

Answer: a) It aids in understanding how the body responds to changes in order to maintain homeostasis. Explanation: Le Chatelier's principle states that a system at equilibrium will react to counteract any change imposed on the system. In the context of human physiology, this principle aids in understanding how the body responds to changes in order to maintain homeostasis.

616. Which of the following is the best example of inductive reasoning?
a) All birds can fly. Penguins are birds. Therefore, penguins can fly.
b) Every time you eat shellfish, you have an allergic reaction. Therefore, you are allergic to shellfish.
c) The moon causes tides. It is a full moon tonight, so there will be high tides.
d) Humans need to breathe to live. You are a human. Therefore, you need to breathe.

Answer: b) Every time you eat shellfish, you have an allergic reaction. Therefore, you are allergic to shellfish. Explanation: Inductive reasoning involves making broad generalizations from specific observations. Here, the observation of an allergic reaction after eating shellfish leads to the general conclusion of a shellfish allergy.

617. A researcher conducts an experiment to test the effectiveness of a new drug. He finds that patients who received the drug showed significant improvement compared to those who did not. However, he later discovers that the patients who received the drug were also undergoing therapy, while those who did not receive the drug were not. This scenario is an example of which flaw in scientific reasoning?
a) Failure to use a control group
b) Confounding variables
c) Selection bias
d) Confirmation bias

Answer: b) Confounding variables. Explanation: Confounding variables are factors outside of the researcher's control that could affect the outcome of an experiment. In this case, the therapy could also have contributed to the patients' improvement, making it hard to attribute the improvement solely to the new drug.

618. Which of the following statements is a hypothesis?
a) Water boils at 100 degrees Celsius at sea level.
b) If I water my plants more, they will grow faster.
c) All swans are white.
d) The Earth revolves around the Sun.

Answer: b) If I water my plants more, they will grow faster. Explanation: A hypothesis is a testable statement or prediction made before carrying out an experiment. In this case, the idea that watering plants more will cause them to grow faster is something that could be tested through an experiment.

619. What is the role of a control group in an experiment?
a) To be exposed to the experimental variable
b) To be used for comparison with the experimental group
c) To confirm the findings of the experimental group
d) To ensure the experiment is ethical

Answer: b) To be used for comparison with the experimental group. Explanation: A control group in an experiment is used as a standard or baseline for comparison. This group is not exposed to the experimental variable, allowing researchers to see what happens without the variable present.

620. In the scientific method, what is the purpose of peer review?
a) To get funding for the research
b) To make the research publicly available
c) To validate and improve the quality of the research
d) To ensure the researchers have followed ethical guidelines

Answer: c) To validate and improve the quality of the research. Explanation: Peer review is an important part of the scientific method, as it allows other experts in the field to evaluate, validate, and provide feedback on the research, thereby ensuring its quality and reliability.

621. A theory differs from a hypothesis in that a theory:
a) Is not testable
b) Is a prediction made before an experiment
c) Is a broad explanation that has been consistently supported by a wide range of evidence
d) Is an observation made after an experiment

Answer: c) Is a broad explanation that has been consistently supported by a wide range of evidence. Explanation: A theory is a well-substantiated explanation of some aspect of the natural world that is acquired through the scientific method and repeatedly tested and confirmed, preferably using a written, pre-defined, protocol of observations and experiments.

622. In a scientific experiment, what is the dependent variable?
a) The variable that the scientist changes
b) The variable that the scientist measures
c) The variable that remains the same throughout the experiment
d) The variable that is not relevant to the experiment

Answer: b) The variable that the scientist measures. Explanation: In a scientific experiment, the dependent variable is the variable being tested or measured. It "depends" on the independent variable, which is the variable being manipulated by the researcher.

623. If a study showed that people who exercise regularly have a lower incidence of heart disease, this would be an example of:
a) An observational study
b) A randomized controlled trial
c) An experimental study
d) A case study

Answer: a) An observational study. Explanation: An observational study observes individuals and measures variables of interest without influencing the responses. In this case, the researchers didn't assign people to exercise or not; they just observed people's regular habits and heart disease incidence.

624. Why is replication important in scientific experiments?
a) It confirms the results of the original experiment
b) It allows the researchers to test multiple variables at once
c) It ensures the ethical conduct of the researchers
d) It helps to get the research published

Answer: a) It confirms the results of the original experiment. Explanation: Replication of experiments is important to verify that the original findings were not due to chance. It increases confidence in the reliability of the result.

625. The placebo effect is a common issue in medical studies. What is one way to control for this effect?
a) Conducting double-blind studies
b) Using a large sample size
c) Only studying serious diseases
d) Ignoring self-reported data from participants

Answer: a) Conducting double-blind studies. Explanation: In a double-blind study, neither the participants nor the researchers know who is receiving the treatment or the placebo. This helps to control for the placebo effect, as participants' and researchers' expectations can't influence the results.

626. Why is the ability to convert between different units of measurement (like kilograms to pounds) important in a healthcare setting?
a) It makes the healthcare professionals look more intelligent.
b) It allows for consistent communication between healthcare providers in different countries.
c) It ensures patients are billed correctly.
d) It is required by healthcare laws.

Answer: b) It allows for consistent communication between healthcare providers in different countries. Explanation: Conversion between units of measurement is important in healthcare to allow for standardized and clear communication about patient care, especially in an increasingly globalized world.

627. In healthcare, why is it crucial to maintain the calibration of measurement tools like scales and thermometers?
a) So they look clean and professional
b) To ensure accurate and reliable measurements
c) Because it's a standard hospital policy
d) To make them last longer

Answer: b) To ensure accurate and reliable measurements. Explanation: Accurate measurements are crucial in healthcare for correct diagnosis and treatment. Calibration ensures measurement tools provide reliable results.

628. The use of microscopes in a healthcare setting primarily helps with what aspect of patient care?
a) Communication with patients
b) Diagnosis of diseases
c) Management of patient records
d) Transportation of patients

Answer: b) Diagnosis of diseases. Explanation: Microscopes are a critical tool in healthcare, particularly in diagnosing diseases. They allow healthcare providers to see cells and microbes that aren't visible to the naked eye, providing critical information for diagnosis.

629. What is the role of a "control" in a healthcare research study?
a) To provide a basis for comparison with the experimental group
b) To act as the group receiving the experimental treatment
c) To oversee the ethical conduct of the research
d) To document and analyze the data from the study

Answer: a) To provide a basis for comparison with the experimental group. Explanation: In a healthcare research study, the control group allows researchers to compare outcomes with the experimental group. This helps to determine the effectiveness of a treatment or intervention.

630. Why is statistical analysis important in healthcare research?
a) It helps in marketing the research to the public
b) It allows for objective evaluation of the data
c) It ensures the personal views of the researchers don't influence the study
d) Both b and c

Answer: d) Both b and c. Explanation: Statistical analysis provides an objective way to interpret data and helps to prevent bias in the interpretation of results. It allows for a clear, objective understanding of the study's findings.

631. In the scientific method, which step directly follows the formation of a hypothesis?
a) Analysis of data
b) Drawing conclusions
c) Performing experiments
d) Gathering background information

Answer: c) Performing experiments. Explanation: After a hypothesis is formulated, the next step in the scientific method is to design and carry out experiments to test the hypothesis.

632. What is the purpose of conducting a "double-blind" study in healthcare research?
a) To protect the privacy of the participants
b) To prevent bias in the interpretation of results
c) To ensure ethical treatment of the participants
d) To control for the placebo effect

Answer: b) To prevent bias in the interpretation of results. Explanation: A double-blind study, where neither the participants nor the researchers know who's in the control or experimental group, helps prevent bias in the study's results. Both the researchers and the participants' expectations can't influence the outcome.

633. In a healthcare experiment, why is it important to only change one variable at a time?
a) To simplify the experimental process
b) To ensure the validity of the results
c) To make it easier to publish the study
d) To make it easier to get ethical approval for the study

Answer: b) To ensure the validity of the results. Explanation: Changing only one variable at a time (the independent variable) allows the researcher to be confident that any changes observed in the dependent variable are due to the variable they manipulated, not some other factor.

634. Why is peer review important in healthcare research?
a) It helps the researchers gain fame in their field
b) It provides a way to share the results with the public
c) It ensures the research is valid and reliable
d) It helps to secure funding for future research

Answer: c) It ensures the research is valid and reliable. Explanation: Peer review involves experts in the same field evaluating the research. This process helps ensure the research is of high quality, the methods are sound, and the conclusions are supported by the data.

635. How can the principles of the scientific method apply to problem-solving in a healthcare setting?
a) By following a protocol without questioning its relevance
b) By applying past experience without considering new information
c) By making a guess about what the problem is and acting on it immediately
d) By observing a problem, formulating a hypothesis, testing it, analyzing the results, and adjusting the approach as needed

Answer: d) By observing a problem, formulating a hypothesis, testing it, analyzing the results, and adjusting the approach as needed. Explanation: The scientific method isn't just for research; it's also a useful problem-solving tool. It involves making careful observations, formulating potential solutions (hypotheses), testing these solutions, analyzing the results, and refining the solutions based on these results.

636. In the process of cellular respiration, what molecule is broken down to produce ATP?
a) Glucose
b) DNA
c) Protein
d) Lipids

Answer: a) Glucose. Explanation: In cellular respiration, glucose is broken down to produce ATP, the cell's primary energy currency. This process involves the steps of glycolysis, the Krebs cycle, and oxidative phosphorylation.

637. What is the primary function of white blood cells in the body?
a) Oxygen transport
b) Blood clotting
c) Immune defense
d) Carrying nutrients

Answer: c) Immune defense. Explanation: White blood cells, or leukocytes, are primarily involved in the body's immune response. They help to defend against pathogens and remove harmful substances from the body.

638. In genetics, what term is used to describe the physical appearance of an organism based on its genotype?
a) Phenotype
b) Genotype
c) Karyotype
d) Allele

Answer: a) Phenotype. Explanation: The phenotype of an organism is the physical manifestation of its genetic information (genotype). This can include traits like eye color, hair color, height, and many others.

639. What is the primary purpose of the scientific method?
a) To win debates
b) To accumulate knowledge
c) To confirm biases
d) To test hypotheses

Answer: d) To test hypotheses. Explanation: The scientific method is a process used to test hypotheses and generate empirical knowledge. It involves observation, hypothesis formulation, experimentation, data analysis, and hypothesis reevaluation.

640. The main function of the mitochondria in a cell is to:
a) Control cell division
b) Protect the cell from damage
c) Produce energy
d) Store genetic information

Answer: c) Produce energy. Explanation: Mitochondria are often referred to as the "powerhouses" of the cell because their primary function is to produce ATP, the cell's main energy currency, through the process of cellular respiration.

641. In which phase of mitosis do the sister chromatids separate?
a) Prophase
b) Metaphase
c) Anaphase
d) Telophase

Answer: c) Anaphase. Explanation: During anaphase, the sister chromatids separate and move towards opposite ends of the cell. This ensures that each new cell will have a complete set of chromosomes.

642. How does DNA replication occur?
a) Conservatively
b) Semi-conservatively
c) Dispersively
d) Randomly

Answer: b) Semi-conservatively. Explanation: DNA replication is semi-conservative, meaning that each of the two new DNA molecules contains one strand from the original DNA molecule and one newly synthesized strand.

643. What's the main difference between eukaryotic and prokaryotic cells?
a) The presence of a cell wall
b) The presence of a nucleus
c) The ability to reproduce
d) The presence of mitochondria

Answer: b) The presence of a nucleus. Explanation: The fundamental difference between eukaryotes and prokaryotes is the presence of a true nucleus in eukaryotes, which houses the cell's DNA. Prokaryotes lack a nucleus and other membrane-bound organelles.

644. Which subatomic particle carries a positive charge?
a) Neutron
b) Electron
c) Proton
d) Quark

Answer: c) Proton. Explanation: In an atom, protons carry a positive charge, neutrons carry no charge (they are neutral), and electrons carry a negative charge.

645. What type of bond involves the sharing of electron pairs between atoms?
a) Ionic bond
b) Covalent bond
c) Hydrogen bond
d) Metallic bond

Answer: b) Covalent bond. Explanation: A covalent bond involves the sharing of one or more pairs of electrons between atoms, allowing each atom to achieve a full outer electron shell and increase its stability. This type of bond often forms between nonmetal atoms.

646. Why do atoms combine to form compounds?
a) To decrease energy
b) To increase energy
c) To maintain energy
d) Energy is not a factor

Answer: a) To decrease energy. Explanation: Atoms combine to form compounds in order to reach a more stable, lower-energy state. Typically, this involves filling their outer electron shells, which is often achieved through the formation of chemical bonds in compounds.

647. How does oxygen contribute to the process of cellular respiration?
a) It's the primary source of energy
b) It acts as a catalyst
c) It accepts electrons and hydrogen ions
d) It donates electrons and hydrogen ions

Answer: c) It accepts electrons and hydrogen ions. Explanation: Oxygen serves as the final electron acceptor in the electron transport chain, a key part of cellular respiration. It accepts electrons and hydrogen ions to form water.

648. What is the main purpose of a control group in an experiment?
a) To validate the results
b) To provide a comparison for the experimental group
c) To manipulate the independent variable
d) To add more data points

Answer: b) To provide a comparison for the experimental group. Explanation: A control group is used as a standard of comparison for the experimental group. It allows researchers to see what happens in the absence of the factor being studied.

649. In the human body, what role does insulin play?
a) It raises blood sugar levels
b) It lowers blood sugar levels
c) It maintains a constant blood sugar level
d) It has no effect on blood sugar levels

Answer: b) It lowers blood sugar levels. Explanation: Insulin is a hormone produced by the pancreas. It helps to regulate blood sugar levels by stimulating the uptake of glucose into cells, thereby lowering blood sugar levels.

650. Why does water have a high heat capacity?
a) It contains a large number of hydrogen bonds
b) It contains a large number of ionic bonds
c) It contains a large number of covalent bonds
d) It contains a large number of metallic bonds

Answer: a) It contains a large number of hydrogen bonds. Explanation: Water's high heat capacity is due to the presence of many hydrogen bonds. These bonds require significant amounts of energy to break, meaning water can absorb a lot of heat before it starts to increase in temperature.

651. What role do ribosomes play in a cell?
a) They synthesize proteins
b) They generate ATP
c) They package and distribute proteins
d) They control cell division

Answer: a) They synthesize proteins. Explanation: Ribosomes are the site of protein synthesis in the cell. They translate the information in mRNA into the amino acid sequence of a protein.

652. What is a common way in which genetic information can be altered?
a) Through mutation
b) Through dehydration
c) Through oxidation
d) Through fermentation

Answer: a) Through mutation. Explanation: Genetic information can be altered through mutation, a process that involves a change in the DNA sequence. Mutations can occur naturally, due to errors in DNA replication, or can be induced by environmental factors.

653. Why is carbon often referred to as the "building block of life"?
a) It's the most abundant element on Earth
b) It forms four bonds
c) It forms ionic bonds
d) It's a liquid at room temperature

Answer: b) It forms four bonds. Explanation: Carbon can form four bonds, which allows it to create complex and diverse structures. This versatility makes it a fundamental element in many biological molecules, including proteins, carbohydrates, lipids, and nucleic acids.

654. What is the purpose of the circulatory system in the human body?
a) To remove waste products from the body
b) To deliver oxygen and nutrients to cells
c) To fight off infections
d) To regulate body temperature

Answer: b) To deliver oxygen and nutrients to cells. Explanation: The main function of the circulatory system is to transport oxygen, nutrients, and other vital substances to cells throughout the body. It also helps to remove waste products.

655. What is the primary role of enzymes in biological systems?
a) They speed up chemical reactions
b) They slow down chemical reactions
c) They stop chemical reactions
d) They have no effect on chemical reactions

Answer: a) They speed up chemical reactions. Explanation: Enzymes are biological catalysts that speed up chemical reactions in cells. They do this by lowering the activation energy required for the reaction to occur.

656. Which element forms the backbone of the macromolecules that make up life: proteins, nucleic acids, carbohydrates, and lipids?
a) Hydrogen
b) Oxygen
c) Carbon
d) Nitrogen

Answer: c) Carbon. Explanation: Carbon's ability to form stable bonds with many elements, including itself, allows it to serve as the structural foundation for many biological molecules.

657. Why is understanding the pH scale important in the healthcare field?
a) It indicates the temperature of a solution
b) It indicates the light absorbance of a solution
c) It indicates the acidity or alkalinity of a solution
d) It indicates the salinity of a solution

Answer: c) It indicates the acidity or alkalinity of a solution. Explanation: In healthcare, monitoring pH can provide crucial information about a patient's health. For example, blood pH can indicate issues like acidosis or alkalosis.

658. How does cell specialization contribute to the functioning of a multicellular organism?
a) It ensures that all cells are identical
b) It allows for a division of labor among cells
c) It increases the chance of cell mutation
d) It prevents cell growth and reproduction

Answer: b) It allows for a division of labor among cells. Explanation: Cell specialization allows cells to perform specific functions efficiently, contributing to the overall functioning and survival of the organism.

659. How does DNA replication ensure the continuity of life?
a) It allows for the creation of energy
b) It provides a blueprint for protein synthesis
c) It guarantees the transmission of genetic information to offspring
d) It assists in the movement of substances across cell membranes

Answer: c) It guarantees the transmission of genetic information to offspring. Explanation: DNA replication copies the genetic information of a cell, ensuring that it can be passed on to the next generation of cells during cell division.

660. Why is homeostasis critical to organismal survival?
a) It allows organisms to change their internal environment frequently
b) It ensures a stable internal environment despite external changes
c) It encourages a constantly changing internal environment
d) It has no impact on an organism's survival

Answer: b) It ensures a stable internal environment despite external changes. Explanation: Homeostasis allows organisms to maintain a relatively stable internal environment, which is crucial for the proper functioning of cells and systems within the body.

661. What is the role of adenosine triphosphate (ATP) in cellular processes?
a) It carries genetic information
b) It provides structural support to the cell
c) It acts as a catalyst for chemical reactions
d) It serves as the main energy currency of the cell

Answer: d) It serves as the main energy currency of the cell. Explanation: ATP is used by cells as a source of energy for many processes, including muscle contraction, nerve impulse propagation, and chemical synthesis.

662. In the context of healthcare, how does an understanding of diffusion apply?
a) It helps understand how blood circulates
b) It explains how nerve signals are transmitted
c) It illustrates how oxygen and nutrients move from blood to tissues
d) It shows how DNA is replicated

Answer: c) It illustrates how oxygen and nutrients move from blood to tissues. Explanation: Understanding diffusion is essential in healthcare because it's the process that facilitates the movement of oxygen, nutrients, and other substances from areas of high concentration to areas of low concentration.

663. What role do carbohydrates play in the body?
a) They provide a source of energy
b) They are a major component of cell membranes
c) They are involved in cell division
d) They play a key role in immune response

Answer: a) They provide a source of energy. Explanation: Carbohydrates are broken down into glucose, which can be used as a primary source of energy by the body's cells.

664. What is the purpose of mitosis in a multicellular organism?
a) It allows for the production of gametes
b) It allows for cell specialization
c) It allows for growth and repair of tissues
d) It allows for digestion of food

Answer: c) It allows for growth and repair of tissues. Explanation: Mitosis is a type of cell division that results in two daughter cells with the same number and kind of chromosomes as the parent nucleus, typically for growth and repair of tissues.

665. How does the understanding of atomic structure apply to drug interactions in the human body?
a) It helps in designing drugs that can interact with specific molecular targets.
b) It helps in understanding the nutritional value of the drug.
c) It explains how drugs are metabolized in the liver.
d) It determines the rate at which a drug is excreted in the urine.

Answer: a) It helps in designing drugs that can interact with specific molecular targets. Explanation: The understanding of atomic structure allows scientists to design drugs that can interact at a molecular level, potentially binding with specific proteins or disrupting certain biological pathways.

666. Which of the following explains why water is essential for life?
a) Water can absorb a high amount of heat, helping regulate body temperature.
b) Water contains carbon, the building block of life.
c) Water is a common solvent for industrial applications.
d) Water is less dense as a solid than a liquid.

Answer: a) Water can absorb a high amount of heat, helping regulate body temperature. Explanation: One of water's many roles in the body includes helping to regulate body temperature. The high specific heat capacity of water allows it to absorb and release heat slowly, preventing sudden temperature changes.

667. Why is understanding cell division important in cancer treatment?
a) It allows for predicting when a person will develop cancer.
b) It helps in understanding the progression and treatment of cancer.
c) It aids in diagnosing psychiatric conditions.
d) It helps in determining a person's genetic traits.

Answer: b) It helps in understanding the progression and treatment of cancer. Explanation: Cancer is characterized by uncontrolled cell division. Understanding this process is crucial to developing treatments that can slow or stop the growth of cancer cells.

668. Why is a pH of 7 considered neutral?
a) It is neither acidic nor basic.
b) It is the average pH of water.
c) It is the pH at which most enzymes function optimally.
d) It is the pH of pure hydrogen.

Answer: a) It is neither acidic nor basic. Explanation: On the pH scale, 7 is considered neutral because it is neither acidic (less than 7) nor basic (greater than 7).

669. How does the structure of DNA relate to its function?
a) The helical structure of DNA allows it to store genetic information.
b) The linear structure of DNA allows it to replicate itself.
c) The circular structure of DNA allows it to produce proteins.
d) The branched structure of DNA allows it to transmit genetic information.

Answer: a) The helical structure of DNA allows it to store genetic information. Explanation: The double helix structure of DNA, with base pairs encoded in the sequence of its strands, allows it to effectively store genetic information.

670. What is the role of the scientific method in healthcare?
a) It provides a systematic way of understanding health conditions and developing treatments.
b) It helps in creating dietary guidelines.
c) It assists in patient communication.
d) It helps in performing surgeries.

Answer: a) It provides a systematic way of understanding health conditions and developing treatments. Explanation: The scientific method, with its focus on observation, hypothesis development, testing, and analysis, is crucial in healthcare research.

671. How do the principles of thermodynamics apply to the human body?
a) They explain how the body gains and loses weight.
b) They determine the structure of the body's cells.
c) They explain how the body maintains its temperature.
d) They determine the body's response to disease.

Answer: c) They explain how the body maintains its temperature. Explanation: Principles of thermodynamics can explain the heat exchange between the body and its environment, contributing to our understanding of how the body maintains a constant internal temperature.

672. How does understanding atomic structure aid in understanding human genetics?
a) It aids in understanding how genes are passed on from parents to offspring.
b) It aids in identifying genetic mutations.
c) It aids in understanding the structure of DNA and genes.
d) It aids in predicting the traits of offspring.

Answer: c) It aids in understanding the structure of DNA and genes. Explanation: Understanding atomic structure helps in understanding the structure and function of DNA and genes, which are composed of atoms.

673. Why is understanding cellular respiration important for healthcare professionals?
a) It allows them to determine how well a patient's cells are producing energy.
b) It allows them to predict a patient's future health.
c) It allows them to diagnose genetic conditions.
d) It allows them to determine a patient's blood type.

Answer: a) It allows them to determine how well a patient's cells are producing energy. Explanation: Cellular respiration is the process by which cells break down glucose and other molecules to produce energy. A disruption in this process can lead to various health problems.

674. Which of the following demonstrates the application of physics in healthcare?
a) The use of MRI technology in diagnosing diseases
b) The use of antibiotics in treating bacterial infections
c) The use of diet in managing diabetes
d) The use of surgery in treating cancer

Answer: a) The use of MRI technology in diagnosing diseases. Explanation: Physics, especially the principles of electromagnetism, play a key role in the functioning of MRI technology. MRI uses a strong magnetic field and radio waves to create detailed images of the body, aiding in disease diagnosis.

675. What is the significance of an understanding of chemical bonds in the healthcare industry?
a) It enables a better understanding of drug interaction at the molecular level.
b) It influences the way in which patients are counseled.
c) It determines how surgeries are performed.
d) It guides the process of hospital administration.

Answer: a) It enables a better understanding of drug interaction at the molecular level. Explanation: An understanding of chemical bonds helps healthcare professionals to predict how drugs will interact at the molecular level, which can influence the efficacy and side effects of medications.

676. Why are radioactive isotopes used in medical imaging techniques like PET scans?
a) They provide a stable and safe source of energy.
b) They help in the creation of three-dimensional images.
c) They emit particles that can be detected to create images of internal structures.
d) They enhance the resolution of the images.

Answer: c) They emit particles that can be detected to create images of internal structures. Explanation: Radioactive isotopes are used because they emit radiation, which can be detected and used to create images of the body's internal structures.

677. How does an understanding of diffusion help healthcare professionals?
a) It helps in the development of effective exercise routines.
b) It helps in understanding how nutrients and waste products are transported in the body.
c) It assists in understanding the psychological aspects of patient care.
d) It helps in the administration of healthcare facilities.

Answer: b) It helps in understanding how nutrients and waste products are transported in the body. Explanation: Diffusion is a key process that enables the transport of substances like nutrients and waste products across cell membranes in the body.

678. What role does pH play in the human body?
a) It helps in determining an individual's genetic makeup.
b) It regulates enzyme activity and biochemical reactions.
c) It determines the physical characteristics of an individual.
d) It aids in the process of digestion.

Answer: b) It regulates enzyme activity and biochemical reactions. Explanation: The pH level in different parts of the body influences enzyme activity and the rate of biochemical reactions, which can affect overall health.

679. Why is an understanding of cellular structure important in healthcare?
a) It helps in the design of hospital infrastructure.
b) It aids in understanding the cause of diseases at a cellular level.
c) It influences the communication strategies with patients.
d) It assists in financial planning in healthcare institutions.

Answer: b) It aids in understanding the cause of diseases at a cellular level. Explanation: Understanding cellular structure is essential to comprehend how cells function normally and how changes in cell structure can lead to disease.

680. What is the role of the scientific method in the diagnosis and treatment of diseases?
a) It provides a systematic way of understanding and treating diseases.
b) It helps in maintaining medical records.
c) It influences the hiring process in healthcare institutions.
d) It aids in the designing of patient wards.

Answer: a) It provides a systematic way of understanding and treating diseases. Explanation: The scientific method provides a systematic and objective approach to discovering how diseases are caused and to developing effective treatments.

681. How does understanding energy transfer help in understanding the functioning of the human body?
a) It explains how cells produce and use energy.
b) It determines how doctors communicate with patients.
c) It helps in designing healthcare policies.
d) It influences how hospitals are administered.

Answer: a) It explains how cells produce and use energy. Explanation: Energy transfer is a key concept in understanding how cells produce and use energy, which is crucial for all bodily functions.

682. In what way is understanding osmosis crucial for healthcare professionals?
a) It helps in the determination of medical insurance policies.
b) It aids in the understanding of fluid balance in the body.
c) It assists in hospital administration.
d) It influences the interior design of healthcare facilities.

Answer: b) It aids in the understanding of fluid balance in the body. Explanation: Osmosis is the process that helps maintain fluid balance in the body. It is a critical concept in understanding various physiological processes and pathologies.

683. How does understanding biological macromolecules aid healthcare professionals?
a) It helps them to develop diet plans for patients.
b) It helps in the development of hospital safety protocols.
c) It helps them in hiring competent staff.
d) It aids in the maintenance of patient records.

Answer: a) It helps them to develop diet plans for patients. Explanation: Understanding biological macromolecules like proteins, carbohydrates, and fats can help healthcare professionals to provide suitable dietary advice to patients.

684. What role does the concept of homeostasis play in healthcare?
a) It influences the way in which healthcare professionals communicate with patients.
b) It helps in the administration of healthcare facilities.
c) It helps in understanding how the body maintains internal balance.
d) It determines how patient data is stored and retrieved.

Answer: c) It helps in understanding how the body maintains internal balance. Explanation: Homeostasis refers to the body's ability to maintain a stable internal environment, despite changes in external conditions. This concept is crucial in understanding how the body functions and how certain medical conditions can disrupt this balance.

685. Why is the understanding of DNA replication important for healthcare professionals?
a) It helps in patient data management.
b) It aids in genetic counseling and understanding hereditary diseases.
c) It assists in the administration of healthcare facilities.
d) It guides the process of hospital construction.

Answer: b) It aids in genetic counseling and understanding hereditary diseases. Explanation: Understanding DNA replication is crucial for healthcare professionals as it plays a major role in understanding genetic diseases, genetic counseling, and personalized medicine.

686. What role does the knowledge of cellular respiration play in healthcare?
a) It aids in hospital administration.
b) It helps in understanding how cells generate energy.
c) It helps in the design of hospital infrastructure.
d) It guides the process of medical billing.

Answer: b) It helps in understanding how cells generate energy. Explanation: Cellular respiration is a set of metabolic reactions that take place in cells of organisms to convert biochemical energy from nutrients into adenosine triphosphate (ATP), which is used by cells for energy.

687. How does understanding phase changes of matter contribute to healthcare?
a) It guides hospital administration policies.
b) It aids in designing hospital infrastructure.
c) It helps in understanding concepts like sterilization and body temperature regulation.
d) It assists in managing patient data.

Answer: c) It helps in understanding concepts like sterilization and body temperature regulation. Explanation: Phase changes of matter underlie several important concepts in healthcare, such as sterilization (where heat changes the state of microbes, killing them) and body temperature regulation.

688. How does understanding the concept of density help in healthcare?
a) It aids in understanding patient dietary requirements.
b) It influences healthcare laws and policies.
c) It guides the process of medical billing.
d) It is crucial in medical imaging and diagnostic techniques.

Answer: d) It is crucial in medical imaging and diagnostic techniques. Explanation: The concept of density is important in several medical imaging techniques, such as ultrasound and CT scans, which rely on differences in density to create images of the body's internal structures.

689. Why is the understanding of acids, bases, and pH important in healthcare?
a) It guides the hiring process in healthcare institutions.
b) It aids in understanding the body's homeostasis and the effect of medications.
c) It helps in the administration of healthcare facilities.
d) It influences the construction of healthcare facilities.

Answer: b) It aids in understanding the body's homeostasis and the effect of medications. Explanation: The body's acid-base balance, or pH, is crucial to numerous biological functions. Disturbances in this balance can lead to health issues. Also, understanding pH is important to know the interaction of certain medications with the body.

690. What role does the concept of pressure play in healthcare?
a) It influences the design of hospital infrastructure.
b) It aids in understanding concepts like blood pressure and the function of respirators.
c) It guides the process of healthcare policy-making.
d) It helps in patient counseling.

Answer: b) It aids in understanding concepts like blood pressure and the function of respirators. Explanation: The concept of pressure is critical in healthcare, with applications ranging from understanding and measuring blood pressure to understanding how respirators function.

691. What is the significance of understanding osmolarity in healthcare?
a) It assists in hospital administration.
b) It aids in understanding fluid and electrolyte balance in the body.
c) It guides the process of healthcare law-making.
d) It helps in the design of hospital infrastructure.

Answer: b) It aids in understanding fluid and electrolyte balance in the body. Explanation: Understanding osmolarity is crucial for healthcare professionals as it helps them understand and manage the body's fluid and electrolyte balance, which can be altered in many diseases.

692. How does the understanding of chemical bonds assist in healthcare?
a) It helps in understanding the structure and function of biological molecules.
b) It assists in the administration of healthcare facilities.
c) It guides the construction of hospital infrastructure.
d) It influences healthcare laws and policies.

Answer: a) It helps in understanding the structure and function of biological molecules. Explanation: Understanding chemical bonds is crucial in healthcare because it forms the basis of the structure and function of biological molecules like DNA, proteins, carbohydrates, and lipids.

693. Why is understanding the properties of water crucial in healthcare?
a) It influences the process of hospital construction.
b) It helps in understanding various biological processes where water plays a crucial role.
c) It guides the process of medical billing.
d) It helps in the management of patient records.

Answer: b) It helps in understanding various biological processes where water plays a crucial role. Explanation: Water is involved in many biological processes, including acting as a solvent, participating in chemical reactions, and assisting in temperature regulation.

694. How does understanding the concept of diffusion help in healthcare?
a) It assists in patient data management.
b) It aids in understanding the movement of drugs and nutrients across cell membranes.
c) It helps in the administration of healthcare facilities.
d) It guides the process of hospital construction.

Answer: b) It aids in understanding the movement of drugs and nutrients across cell membranes. Explanation: Diffusion is a fundamental concept in healthcare, underlying the way in which drugs and nutrients move across cell membranes, among other things.

695. How does knowledge about the particle nature of matter assist in healthcare?
a) It aids in developing and executing marketing strategies for hospitals.
b) It assists in designing the structure of healthcare facilities.
c) It helps in understanding the behavior of pharmaceuticals at the molecular level.
d) It guides the process of maintaining hospital records.

Answer: c) It helps in understanding the behavior of pharmaceuticals at the molecular level. Explanation: The particle nature of matter is fundamental to understanding how pharmaceuticals interact at the molecular level, influencing their efficacy and potential side effects.

696. Why is understanding the concept of gas laws significant in healthcare?
a) It assists in creating hospital administration policies.
b) It aids in the understanding of respiration and the administration of anesthetics.
c) It helps in maintaining patient records.
d) It guides the process of medical billing.

Answer: b) It aids in the understanding of respiration and the administration of anesthetics. Explanation: Gas laws are essential to understanding how gases behave under varying conditions, which is fundamental to areas like respiration and the administration of gaseous anesthetics.

697. How does understanding the concept of isotopes contribute to healthcare?
a) It aids in medical imaging and cancer treatment.
b) It guides hospital administration processes.
c) It assists in maintaining patient data.
d) It influences healthcare laws and policies.

Answer: a) It aids in medical imaging and cancer treatment. Explanation: Isotopes, especially radioactive ones, play a key role in medical imaging techniques like PET scans. Additionally, some isotopes are used in cancer treatment, like radioactive iodine for thyroid cancer.

698. What role does the understanding of thermodynamics play in healthcare?
a) It helps in understanding how the human body exchanges energy with its environment.
b) It assists in designing hospital infrastructure.
c) It aids in creating healthcare laws and policies.
d) It guides the process of patient counseling.

Answer: a) It helps in understanding how the human body exchanges energy with its environment. Explanation: Thermodynamics is fundamental to understanding how the human body exchanges energy with its surroundings, an essential aspect of metabolism, body temperature regulation, and more.

699. How does knowledge about the electromagnetic spectrum contribute to healthcare?
a) It assists in the construction of healthcare facilities.
b) It aids in understanding and utilizing medical imaging technologies.
c) It guides the hiring process in healthcare institutions.
d) It influences healthcare marketing strategies.

Answer: b) It aids in understanding and utilizing medical imaging technologies. Explanation: Different parts of the electromagnetic spectrum are used in different medical imaging technologies, like X-rays, MRIs, and ultrasounds.

700. Why is understanding of chemical equilibrium important in healthcare?
a) It helps in understanding how reactions proceed in the body.
b) It assists in hospital administration.
c) It aids in healthcare policy making.
d) It guides the process of medical billing.

Answer: a) It helps in understanding how reactions proceed in the body. Explanation: Chemical equilibrium is a state where the rate of the forward reaction equals the rate of the backward reaction. In the human body, many reactions are in a state of dynamic equilibrium, which is critical to maintaining homeostasis.

701. How does the knowledge of the periodic table assist in healthcare?
a) It helps in understanding the properties of elements used in medications.
b) It guides the construction of healthcare facilities.
c) It aids in maintaining patient records.
d) It assists in healthcare law-making.

Answer: a) It helps in understanding the properties of elements used in medications. Explanation: The periodic table organizes elements by their properties, which is fundamental to understanding the behavior of elements used in medications and biological processes.

702. What role does the understanding of acid-base balance play in healthcare?
a) It helps in understanding human physiology and pathology.
b) It aids in hospital infrastructure planning.
c) It guides the process of medical billing.
d) It assists in designing healthcare policies and laws.

Answer: a) It helps in understanding human physiology and pathology. Explanation: Acid-base balance is crucial to maintaining the body's pH levels within a narrow range, which is necessary for enzymatic reactions and overall human physiology. Disruptions in this balance can lead to pathologies.

703. How does the knowledge of covalent bonding assist in healthcare?
a) It aids in medical imaging interpretation.
b) It assists in understanding the structure of complex biological molecules.
c) It guides the administration process in healthcare institutions.
d) It influences the creation of healthcare laws and policies.

Answer: b) It assists in understanding the structure of complex biological molecules. Explanation: Covalent bonds are a key aspect of the structure of complex biological molecules such as DNA, proteins, and fats. Understanding this helps us understand their function and behavior in the body.

704. Why is understanding the properties of water significant in healthcare?
a) It helps in designing hospital uniforms.
b) It aids in understanding the principles of human hydration and cellular function.
c) It assists in medical billing.
d) It guides the construction of healthcare facilities.

Answer: b) It aids in understanding the principles of human hydration and cellular function. Explanation: Water's unique properties make it vital for human hydration, maintaining body temperature, and enabling many cellular functions, including transportation of nutrients and waste.

705. How does knowledge about the Doppler effect contribute to healthcare?
a) It aids in the interpretation of echocardiograms and other ultrasound techniques.
b) It assists in creating healthcare marketing strategies.
c) It helps in designing healthcare facilities.
d) It guides the maintenance of hospital records.

Answer: a) It aids in the interpretation of echocardiograms and other ultrasound techniques. Explanation: The Doppler effect is used in ultrasound techniques, including echocardiograms, to monitor the movement of blood and detect abnormalities.

706. How does an understanding of diffusion contribute to healthcare?
a) It aids in understanding how substances move across cell membranes.
b) It guides the hospital administration process.
c) It assists in maintaining patient records.
d) It influences healthcare laws and policies.

Answer: a) It aids in understanding how substances move across cell membranes. Explanation: Diffusion is a process by which molecules move from an area of higher concentration to one of lower concentration. This principle is fundamental to understanding how gases like oxygen and carbon dioxide, or nutrients, are exchanged in cells.

707. Why is understanding the concept of concentration gradients important in healthcare?
a) It helps in understanding how substances move in the body.
b) It assists in hospital administration.
c) It aids in creating healthcare laws and policies.
d) It guides the process of medical billing.

Answer: a) It helps in understanding how substances move in the body. Explanation: A concentration gradient is a change in the concentration of a substance across a space. Understanding this concept is critical for understanding how substances are transported in the body, including the delivery of nutrients to cells and the removal of waste products.

708. How does knowledge about the electron transport chain assist in healthcare?
a) It helps in understanding the process of energy production in the body.
b) It guides hospital administration processes.
c) It assists in maintaining patient data.
d) It influences healthcare laws and policies.

Answer: a) It helps in understanding the process of energy production in the body. Explanation: The electron transport chain is a part of cellular respiration, a process that converts biochemical energy from nutrients into adenosine triphosphate (ATP

709. What is the function of ribosomes in a cell?"
a) They aid in cell division.
b) They synthesize proteins.
c) They are responsible for energy production.
d) They act as the cell's waste disposal system.

Answer: b) They synthesize proteins. Explanation: Ribosomes are small organelles within a cell that play a key role in the process of protein synthesis, translating mRNA into proteins, a process called translation.

710. What type of bond is formed between nitrogenous bases in DNA?
a) Ionic bond
b) Covalent bond
c) Hydrogen bond
d) Van der Waals forces

Answer: c) Hydrogen bond. Explanation: Nitrogenous bases in DNA are linked together by hydrogen bonds, which contribute to the double helix structure of DNA.

711. What is the correct sequence in which inhaled air passes through the respiratory tract?
a) Trachea -> bronchi -> bronchioles -> alveoli
b) Alveoli -> bronchioles -> bronchi -> trachea
c) Bronchi -> trachea -> bronchioles -> alveoli
d) Bronchioles -> bronchi -> trachea -> alveoli

Answer: a) Trachea -> bronchi -> bronchioles -> alveoli. Explanation: This is the correct sequence for the passage of air during inhalation. The air travels down the trachea, divides into the bronchi, further divides into bronchioles, and finally reaches the alveoli where gas exchange occurs.

712. Why is understanding the concept of anatomical position crucial in healthcare?
a) It aids in the proper administration of medications.
b) It provides a standardized point of reference in describing the human body.
c) It helps in understanding the genetic basis of diseases.
d) It guides the process of medical billing.

Answer: b) It provides a standardized point of reference in describing the human body. Explanation: The anatomical position is a standardized method of viewing the body, used as a reference in medicine to describe the locations of structures, locations, or directional terms.

713. Which of the following statements is true about hydrogen bonds?
a) They are the strongest type of chemical bond.
b) They are responsible for the double helix structure of DNA.
c) They can only occur between hydrogen and oxygen.
d) They are responsible for covalent bonding in water.

Answer: b) They are responsible for the double helix structure of DNA. Explanation: Hydrogen bonds are a type of weak bond that form between a hydrogen atom in one molecule and another atom, often oxygen or nitrogen, in another molecule. They play a crucial role in giving DNA its characteristic double helix shape.

714. What is the basic building block of proteins?
a) Amino acids
b) Nucleic acids
c) Saccharides
d) Lipids

Answer: a) Amino acids. Proteins are made up of chains of amino acids linked together by peptide bonds. They perform a vast array of functions within organisms including catalyzing metabolic reactions, DNA replication, responding to stimuli, and transporting molecules from one location to another.

715. What is the primary role of insulin in the body?
a) Breaks down glucose for energy
b) Stimulates the uptake of glucose into cells
c) Increases blood glucose levels
d) Converts proteins to glucose

Answer: b) Stimulates the uptake of glucose into cells. Insulin is a hormone produced by the pancreas that allows cells in the body to take in glucose and use it for energy.

716. What is the main component of the human body's first line of defense against pathogens?
a) Skin
b) White blood cells
c) Antibodies
d) Platelets

Answer: a) Skin. The skin acts as a physical barrier against pathogens, preventing them from entering the body. Other elements of the first line of defense include mucous membranes and secretions like sweat and tears.

717. What is the main function of the large intestine in the digestive system?
a) Digestion of food
b) Absorption of nutrients
c) Absorption of water
d) Production of bile

Answer: c) Absorption of water. The large intestine, or colon, primarily absorbs water and electrolytes from the remaining indigestible food matter, and transmits the useless waste material from the body.

718. Which hormone is primarily responsible for the regulation of the metabolic rate?
a) Insulin
b) Thyroxine
c) Glucagon
d) Estrogen

Answer: b) Thyroxine. The thyroid gland produces the hormone thyroxine, which plays a crucial role in heart and digestive function, metabolism, brain development, bone health, and muscle control.

719. What is the primary function of DNA?
a) Provides energy for cells
b) Regulates the cell cycle
c) Stores and transmits genetic information
d) Produces proteins

Answer: c) Stores and transmits genetic information. DNA is a molecule that carries most of the genetic instructions used in the development, functioning, and reproduction of all known living organisms and many viruses.

720. What is the role of chloroplasts in plant cells?
a) Energy production
b) Protein synthesis
c) Genetic material storage
d) Waste disposal

Answer: a) Energy production. Chloroplasts are the site of photosynthesis, a process where plants convert light energy into chemical energy in the form of glucose.

721. What is a characteristic of malignant tumors?
a) They grow slowly and remain localized
b) They can invade surrounding tissues and spread to other parts of the body
c) They are usually harmless
d) They do not lead to cancer

Answer: b) They can invade surrounding tissues and spread to other parts of the body. Malignant tumors are cancerous and can spread aggressively throughout the body through the blood or lymphatic system.

722. What is the primary role of leukocytes (white blood cells) in the human body?
a) Carry oxygen to tissues
b) Coagulate blood to prevent bleeding
c) Fight infection and disease
d) Transport waste products

Answer: c) Fight infection and disease. White blood cells are a key component of the immune system and help to defend the body against both infectious disease and foreign materials.

723. Which of the following best describes homeostasis?
a) The process by which organisms maintain a relatively stable internal environment.
b) The tendency of an organism to change in response to the environment.
c) The development of complex structures from simpler ones.
d) The ability of an organism to repair itself.

Answer: a) The process by which organisms maintain a relatively stable internal environment. Homeostasis involves maintaining the balance in the body's internal environment, allowing it to function optimally despite external changes.

724. Which of the following is an example of a chemical change?
a) Melting ice
b) Dissolving sugar in water
c) Burning wood
d) Cutting paper

Answer: c) Burning wood. Chemical changes involve a process where the substance's molecular structure changes. Burning wood is an example of a chemical change because it involves combustion, a process that produces new substances: ash, smoke, and gases.

725. Which of the following molecules is a primary source of quick, accessible energy for cells?
a) DNA
b) Lipids
c) Proteins
d) Glucose

Answer: d) Glucose. Glucose is a simple sugar that is an important energy source in living organisms and is a component of many carbohydrates.

726. Which of the following is not a component of Darwin's theory of natural selection?
a) Inheritance
b) Overproduction
c) Design and purpose
d) Variation

Answer: c) Design and purpose. Darwin's theory of natural selection describes the process by which species evolve over time through a process of natural selection. It does not involve a predetermined design or purpose.

727. In the context of genetics, what is a phenotype?
a) The genetic makeup of an organism
b) The physical characteristics of an organism
c) The potential traits an organism can inherit
d) The variations in a gene pool

Answer: b) The physical characteristics of an organism. A phenotype refers to the observable characteristics or traits of an organism that are determined by its genetic makeup and environmental influences.

728. What does an atomic number represent?
a) The number of neutrons in an atom
b) The number of electrons in an atom
c) The number of protons in an atom
d) The number of isotopes in an atom

Answer: c) The number of protons in an atom. The atomic number is the number of protons in the nucleus of an atom, which determines the chemical properties of an element and its place in the periodic table.

729. What is the role of the mitochondria in eukaryotic cells?
a) Photosynthesis
b) Protein synthesis
c) Energy production
d) Digestion of nutrients

Answer: c) Energy production. Mitochondria are known as the "powerhouses" of the cell. They are responsible for producing adenosine triphosphate (ATP), the cell's main source of energy.

730. What is the primary function of the respiratory system?
a) To deliver oxygen to the body's cells
b) To remove waste from the bloodstream
c) To circulate blood throughout the body
d) To control body temperature

Answer: a) To deliver oxygen to the body's cells. The respiratory system is responsible for inhaling oxygen and exhaling carbon dioxide. The oxygen is then transported to cells throughout the body via the circulatory system.

731. Which of the following is a main function of the nervous system?
a) To provide structural support
b) To control and coordinate body functions
c) To transport nutrients and oxygen
d) To protect the body from infection

Answer: b) To control and coordinate body functions. The nervous system receives sensory input, interprets and integrates this information, and then coordinates voluntary and involuntary responses.

732. What is the process by which plants convert light energy into chemical energy?
a) Cellular respiration
b) Mitosis
c) Fermentation
d) Photosynthesis

Answer: d) Photosynthesis. Photosynthesis is the process by which green plants, algae, and certain bacteria transform light energy, usually from the sun, into chemical energy in the form of glucose or other sugars.

733. How is osmosis different from diffusion?
a) Osmosis requires energy, while diffusion does not.
b) Osmosis is the movement of water, while diffusion involves any type of molecule.
c) Osmosis only happens in living cells, while diffusion can occur anywhere.
d) Osmosis can't happen through semi-permeable membranes, while diffusion can.

Answer: b) Osmosis is the movement of water, while diffusion involves any type of molecule. Osmosis specifically refers to the movement of water across a semi-permeable membrane from an area of lower solute concentration to an area of higher solute concentration.

734. Which of the following best describes the function of white blood cells?
a) They deliver oxygen to tissues.
b) They clot blood to prevent excessive bleeding.
c) They fight off foreign invaders in the body.
d) They transport nutrients to cells.

Answer: c) They fight off foreign invaders in the body. White blood cells, or leukocytes, play a critical role in the body's immune response and are essential for warding off infections and diseases.

735. What is the role of enzymes in metabolic reactions?
a) They decrease the rate of the reactions.
b) They increase the activation energy needed for the reactions.
c) They act as catalysts to speed up the reactions.
d) They create new molecules during the reactions.

Answer: c) They act as catalysts to speed up the reactions. Enzymes are biological catalysts that increase the speed of chemical reactions in the body without being consumed in the process.

736. What type of bond is responsible for holding the two strands of DNA's double helix together?
a) Ionic bond
b) Covalent bond
c) Hydrogen bond
d) Van der Waals bond

Answer: c) Hydrogen bond. Hydrogen bonds occur between the nitrogenous bases of the two DNA strands, holding them together and contributing to the double helix structure.

737. How do isotopes of the same element differ from each other?
a) In the number of protons
b) In the number of electrons
c) In the number of neutrons
d) In the type of bonds they form

Answer: c) In the number of neutrons. Isotopes of an element have the same number of protons (and therefore the same atomic number), but different numbers of neutrons.

738. What is the primary function of the lymphatic system?
a) To regulate body temperature
b) To circulate oxygenated blood
c) To produce hormones for body regulation
d) To defend the body against disease

Answer: d) To defend the body against disease. The lymphatic system contributes to the body's immune defenses and helps in the removal and filtration of interstitial fluid from tissues.

739. What is the primary structure responsible for ATP production in animal cells?
a) Nucleus
b) Ribosome
c) Mitochondrion
d) Endoplasmic reticulum

Answer: c) Mitochondrion. Mitochondria, often referred to as the "powerhouses" of the cell, are the primary sites of ATP production in animal cells.

740. How does a catalyst affect the activation energy of a reaction?
a) It increases the activation energy.
b) It decreases the activation energy.
c) It has no effect on the activation energy.
d) It changes the activation energy unpredictably.

Answer: b) It decreases the activation energy. A catalyst speeds up a chemical reaction by lowering the activation energy, which is the energy needed to initiate the reaction.

741. In which part of a plant cell does photosynthesis primarily occur?
a) Nucleus
b) Mitochondria
c) Chloroplasts
d) Ribosomes

Answer: c) Chloroplasts. Chloroplasts contain chlorophyll, the pigment responsible for absorbing light energy for photosynthesis.

742. Why does water have a high specific heat capacity?
a) It doesn't have a high specific heat capacity.
b) It is a product of combustion reactions.
c) Its molecules can form hydrogen bonds with each other.
d) Its molecular structure allows it to rotate easily.

Answer: c) Its molecules can form hydrogen bonds with each other. This unique property allows water to absorb and store a large amount of heat energy without a significant change in its temperature.

743. Which of the following types of cells are found in the brain?
a) Myocytes
b) Neurons
c) Erythrocytes
d) Hepatocytes

Answer: b) Neurons. Neurons, or nerve cells, are the key players in the brain and the nervous system. They transmit information to other nerve cells, muscle, or gland cells.

744. What are carbohydrates composed of?
a) Carbon, hydrogen, and nitrogen
b) Carbon, hydrogen, and oxygen
c) Carbon, oxygen, and nitrogen
d) Carbon, hydrogen, and phosphorus

Answer: b) Carbon, hydrogen, and oxygen. Carbohydrates are organic compounds made up of carbon, hydrogen, and oxygen atoms.

745. Which organ in the human body produces insulin?
a) Heart
b) Pancreas
c) Liver
d) Kidney

Answer: b) Pancreas. The pancreas is responsible for producing insulin, a hormone that regulates blood sugar levels.

746. What is the term for a chemical reaction in which electrons are lost?
a) Reduction
b) Oxidation
c) Hydrolysis
d) Esterification

Answer: b) Oxidation. Oxidation is the loss of electrons during a reaction by a molecule, atom, or ion.

747. Which structure of the heart contains the body's natural pacemaker?
a) Left atrium
b) Right atrium
c) Left ventricle
d) Right ventricle

Answer: b) Right atrium. The sinoatrial (SA) node, located in the right atrium of the heart, acts as the natural pacemaker.

748. What is the powerhouse of the cell, known for energy production?
a) Nucleus
b) Ribosome
c) Mitochondria
d) Endoplasmic Reticulum

Answer: c) Mitochondria. Often referred to as the "powerhouses" of the cell, mitochondria are responsible for producing ATP, the main energy currency of cells.

749. How many chromosomes does a human somatic cell have?
a) 23
b) 46
c) 69
d) 92

Answer: b) 46. A typical human somatic (body) cell contains 46 chromosomes: 23 pairs, one of each pair inherited from each parent.

750. What is the primary function of the respiratory system?
a) To deliver nutrients to the body
b) To eliminate waste from the body
c) To exchange gases with the environment
d) To circulate blood throughout the body

Answer: c) To exchange gases with the environment. The respiratory system allows the body to take in oxygen and expel carbon dioxide, a process known as gas exchange.

751. What role does DNA polymerase play in DNA replication?
a) It unzips the double helix structure.
b) It adds nucleotides to the growing DNA strand.
c) It seals the gaps between the Okazaki fragments.
d) It repairs mistakes in the DNA sequence.

Answer: b) It adds nucleotides to the growing DNA strand. DNA polymerase is the main enzyme involved in DNA replication, and its primary role is to add new nucleotides to the growing DNA strand.

752. Which of the following is not one of the four main types of tissues in the human body?
a) Connective
b) Muscular
c) Endocrine
d) Epithelial

Answer: c) Endocrine. The four main types of tissues are epithelial, connective, muscle, and nervous tissue. The endocrine system is a group of glands and parts of glands that produce hormones, but it's not a type of tissue.

753. Which part of the cell is responsible for breaking down waste products?
a) Nucleus
b) Lysosome
c) Ribosome
d) Mitochondria

Answer: b) Lysosome. Lysosomes are responsible for breaking down waste products in the cell and are often referred to as the cell's recycling center.

754. What is the atomic number of an element determined by?
a) Number of protons
b) Number of neutrons
c) Number of electrons
d) Number of isotopes

Answer: a) Number of protons. The atomic number of an element is determined by the number of protons in the nucleus of an atom.

755. What are the building blocks of proteins?
a) Nucleotides
b) Amino acids
c) Fatty acids
d) Monosaccharides

Answer: b) Amino acids. Proteins are made up of amino acids, which are linked together in a specific sequence.

756. What type of joint allows for rotation, such as turning the head side to side?
a) Hinge joint
b) Pivot joint
c) Saddle joint
d) Ball and socket joint

Answer: b) Pivot joint. A pivot joint allows for rotation, and one example in the body is the joint between the first and second vertebrae, which allows for turning the head.

757. What is the primary function of the circulatory system?
a) To provide structure to the body
b) To carry oxygen and nutrients to cells
c) To protect the body from disease
d) To remove waste from the body

Answer: b) To carry oxygen and nutrients to cells. The circulatory system's primary function is to transport oxygen, nutrients, and other substances throughout the body.

758. Which phase of mitosis is characterized by the alignment of chromosomes along the center of the cell?
a) Prophase
b) Metaphase
c) Anaphase
d) Telophase

Answer: b) Metaphase. During metaphase, the chromosomes line up along the middle of the cell.

759. Which organ system is responsible for removing waste from the body?
a) Digestive system
b) Respiratory system
c) Excretory system
d) Circulatory system

Answer: c) Excretory system. The excretory system is primarily responsible for the removal of waste and toxins from the body.

760. Which of the following is an example of a covalent bond?
a) Sodium chloride
b) Water
c) Calcium fluoride
d) Potassium iodide

Answer: b) Water. In water (H2O), the hydrogen and oxygen atoms are bonded together by covalent bonds.

761. Which layer of the skin contains sweat glands?
a) Epidermis
b) Dermis
c) Subcutaneous
d) Stratum corneum

Answer: b) Dermis. The dermis layer of the skin contains sweat glands, as well as nerves and blood vessels.

762. What is the term for the variable in an experiment that is being measured?
a) Control variable
b) Independent variable
c) Dependent variable
d) Confounding variable

Answer: c) Dependent variable. In an experiment, the dependent variable is what is being measured or tested, while the independent variable is what is being manipulated or changed.

763. Which type of cell division results in two identical daughter cells?
a) Mitosis
b) Meiosis
c) Binary fission
d) Fragmentation

Answer: a) Mitosis. Mitosis is the process by which a cell divides into two identical daughter cells, each with the same number of chromosomes as the parent cell.

764. What is the term for a substance that cannot be broken down into simpler substances by chemical means?
a) Compound
b) Element
c) Molecule
d) Isotope

Answer: b) Element. An element is a substance that cannot be broken down into simpler substances by chemical reactions.

765. Which organ in the human body produces insulin?
a) Liver
b) Pancreas
c) Kidneys
d) Stomach

Answer: b) Pancreas. The pancreas produces insulin, a hormone that regulates blood glucose levels.

766. What type of bond is formed when electrons are transferred from one atom to another?
a) Covalent bond
b) Hydrogen bond
c) Ionic bond
d) Metallic bond

Answer: c) Ionic bond. An ionic bond is formed when one atom transfers one or more electrons to another atom.

767. Which part of the brain is responsible for coordinating voluntary movements and balance?
a) Cerebrum
b) Cerebellum
c) Brainstem
d) Hypothalamus

Answer: b) Cerebellum. The cerebellum is responsible for coordinating voluntary movements and maintaining posture and balance.

768. In genetics, what does the term "phenotype" refer to?
a) The genetic makeup of an organism
b) The physical characteristics of an organism
c) The potential traits an organism can pass on to its offspring
d) The process of DNA replication

Answer: b) The physical characteristics of an organism. Phenotype refers to the physical characteristics of an organism that are a result of the interaction of its genotype with the environment.

769. What is the name of the process by which plants convert light energy into chemical energy?
a) Cellular respiration
b) Fermentation
c) Photosynthesis
d) Digestion

Answer: c) Photosynthesis. Photosynthesis is the process by which plants convert light energy into chemical energy, which is stored in the bonds of glucose.

770. In a solution, what is the term for the substance that is being dissolved?
a) Solvent
b) Solute
c) Solution
d) Suspension

Answer: b) Solute. In a solution, the solute is the substance that is being dissolved by the solvent.

771. Which of the following best describes the function of white blood cells?
a) They carry oxygen to body tissues.
b) They clot blood to prevent excessive bleeding.
c) They fight off infections and diseases.
d) They regulate body temperature.

Answer: c) They fight off infections and diseases. White blood cells, or leukocytes, are primarily involved in the body's immune response against infections and diseases.

772. When conducting an experiment, why is it important to have a control group?
a) To ensure all variables are kept constant
b) To have a standard for comparison with the experimental group
c) To eliminate the possibility of confounding variables
d) To ensure the experiment is ethical

Answer: b) To have a standard for comparison with the experimental group. A control group is used in an experiment as a standard of comparison for the experimental group, allowing researchers to determine the effect of the variable being tested.

773. What type of macromolecule is an enzyme?
a) Protein
b) Carbohydrate
c) Lipid
d) Nucleic acid

Answer: a) Protein. Enzymes are proteins that catalyze chemical reactions in living organisms.

774. Which of the following best describes the primary function of the respiratory system?
a) Regulate body temperature
b) Transport nutrients to cells
c) Facilitate gas exchange
d) Remove waste from the bloodstream

Answer: c) Facilitate gas exchange. The primary function of the respiratory system is to facilitate gas exchange, providing oxygen to the body's cells and removing carbon dioxide.

775. Which of the following best describes the role of a catalyst in a chemical reaction?
a) Increases the temperature of the reaction
b) Changes the direction of the reaction
c) Increases the rate of the reaction
d) Creates new products in the reaction

Answer: c) Increases the rate of the reaction. A catalyst speeds up a chemical reaction by lowering the energy needed for the reaction to proceed.

776. What is the main function of the nervous system?
a) Control body movement and coordination
b) Transport blood and nutrients throughout the body
c) Protect the body from disease
d) Detect and interpret information from the environment

Answer: d) Detect and interpret information from the environment. The nervous system's main function is to detect, transmit, and process information from the environment, and coordinate bodily functions based on this information.

777. In terms of genetics, what is a recessive trait?
a) A trait that always shows up in the offspring
b) A trait that only shows up when two copies of the gene are present
c) A trait that is dominant over all other traits
d) A trait that can be passed on to offspring but does not show up

Answer: b) A trait that only shows up when two copies of the gene are present. A recessive trait is a characteristic that appears in an individual only if two copies of the gene that codes for the trait are present.

778. What type of reaction occurs when a molecule is broken down into smaller components?
a) Synthesis reaction
b) Decomposition reaction
c) Single replacement reaction
d) Neutralization reaction

Answer: b) Decomposition reaction. A decomposition reaction occurs when a compound is broken down into smaller components.

779. What type of muscle is found in the walls of organs and structures like the esophagus and blood vessels?
a) Skeletal muscle
b) Cardiac muscle
c) Smooth muscle
d) Connective muscle

Answer: c) Smooth muscle. Smooth muscle, which is involuntary, is found in the walls of organs and structures like the esophagus and blood vessels.

780. Which of the following is a major function of the circulatory system?
a) Synthesizing hormones
b) Removing waste products from the body
c) Producing body movement
d) Delivering oxygen and nutrients to the cells

Answer: d) Delivering oxygen and nutrients to the cells. The circulatory system, also known as the cardiovascular system, is primarily responsible for the transportation of oxygen, nutrients, and hormones to cells throughout the body.

781. Which of the following is a key principle of the scientific method?
a) Ideas must be tested through experimentation
b) Conclusions should be based on personal beliefs
c) Hypotheses cannot be revised
d) Scientific investigations do not need to be repeated

Answer: a) Ideas must be tested through experimentation. A fundamental principle of the scientific method is that ideas and hypotheses must be empirically tested through experimentation and observation.

782. What is the term for a change in a DNA sequence that affects genetic information?
a) Mutation
b) Translation
c) Transcription
d) Replication

Answer: a) Mutation. A mutation is a change in a DNA sequence that can affect genetic information and potentially lead to the production of a protein with a different structure or function.

783. Which term describes the movement of water molecules from an area of higher concentration to an area of lower concentration?
a) Diffusion
b) Osmosis
c) Active transport
d) Endocytosis

Answer: b) Osmosis. Osmosis is the movement of water across a semipermeable membrane from an area of higher water concentration to an area of lower water concentration.

784. What is the function of mitochondria in cells?
a) Protein synthesis
b) Energy production
c) DNA storage
d) Waste removal

Answer: b) Energy production. Mitochondria are often referred to as the "powerhouses" of the cell because they produce ATP (adenosine triphosphate), the cell's main energy-carrying molecule.

785. What is the role of ribosomes in a cell?
a) DNA replication
b) Protein synthesis
c) Energy production
d) Cell division

Answer: b) Protein synthesis. Ribosomes are the sites of protein synthesis in the cell, translating genetic information in the form of mRNA into proteins.

786. In what part of the cell does DNA replication occur?
a) Nucleus
b) Mitochondria
c) Cytoplasm
d) Endoplasmic reticulum

Answer: a) Nucleus. DNA replication occurs in the nucleus of a cell where the cell's genetic material is stored.

787. What is the main structural difference between DNA and RNA?
a) Number of strands
b) Type of sugar
c) Presence of a phosphate group
d) Both a) and b)

Answer: d) Both a) and b). DNA is double-stranded and contains deoxyribose sugar, while RNA is single-stranded and contains ribose sugar.

788. What is the main function of the lymphatic system?
a) To produce hormones
b) To digest food
c) To defend the body against disease
d) To control body temperature

Answer: c) To defend the body against disease. The lymphatic system plays a key role in the immune response, helping to defend the body against disease by producing and transporting white blood cells and by removing foreign substances from the blood and lymph.

789. Which element is necessary for the proper functioning of the thyroid gland?
a) Iron
b) Calcium
c) Potassium
d) Iodine

Answer: d) Iodine. The thyroid gland uses iodine to make thyroid hormones, which regulate metabolism.

790. What is the main role of the kidney in the human body?
a) To filter the blood and remove waste
b) To produce and release hormones
c) To control breathing
d) To regulate body temperature

Answer: a) To filter the blood and remove waste. The kidneys are responsible for filtering the blood, removing waste products and excess substances, and regulating the balance of electrolytes in the body.

791. What is the main function of the Golgi apparatus in a cell?
a) To produce energy
b) To synthesize proteins
c) To package and distribute proteins and lipids
d) To store DNA

Answer: c) To package and distribute proteins and lipids. The Golgi apparatus modifies, sorts, and packages proteins and lipids for transport to their intended destinations within or outside the cell.

792. What is the pH of a neutral solution?
a) 0
b) 7
c) 14
d) 21

Answer: b) 7. On the pH scale, which ranges from 0 to 14, a pH of 7 represents a neutral solution. Acidic solutions have a pH less than 7, while basic or alkaline solutions have a pH greater than 7.

793. What are antigens?
a) Cells that protect the body against pathogens
b) Proteins that antibodies bind to
c) White blood cells
d) Foreign substances that trigger an immune response

Answer: d) Foreign substances that trigger an immune response. Antigens are typically foreign substances, such as bacteria and viruses, that trigger an immune response in the body.

794. What role does calcium play in muscle contraction?
a) It blocks the binding sites on actin
b) It binds to troponin and triggers the movement of tropomyosin
c) It breaks the link between myosin and actin
d) It is necessary for the release of acetylcholine at the neuromuscular junction

Answer: b) It binds to troponin and triggers the movement of tropomyosin. When calcium binds to troponin, it causes a shift in tropomyosin, exposing binding sites for myosin on the actin filament, which enables muscle contraction.

795. What type of biological molecule are enzymes?
a) Carbohydrates
b) Lipids
c) Proteins
d) Nucleic acids

Answer: c) Proteins. Enzymes are proteins that act as catalysts to speed up chemical reactions in the body.

796. What is the term for the minimum amount of energy required to start a chemical reaction?
a) Activation energy
b) Kinetic energy
c) Potential energy
d) Thermal energy

Answer: a) Activation energy. Activation energy is the minimum energy required to initiate a chemical reaction.

797. Which hormone is primarily responsible for the regulation of the metabolic rate?
a) Insulin
b) Glucagon
c) Thyroxine
d) Cortisol

Answer: c) Thyroxine. Thyroxine, also known as T4, is a hormone produced by the thyroid gland. It plays a key role in regulating the body's metabolic rate.

798. What is the role of the medulla oblongata in the human body?
a) It controls voluntary muscle movements
b) It controls balance and coordination
c) It regulates heart rate, breathing, and blood pressure
d) It regulates body temperature

Answer: c) It regulates heart rate, breathing, and blood pressure. The medulla oblongata is a part of the brainstem that plays a crucial role in the autonomic (involuntary) control of heart rate, breathing, and blood pressure.

799. Which of the following sentences demonstrates correct subject-verb agreement?
a) The pack of wolves are howling at the moon.
b) Neither of the cats likes to play with toys.
c) The group of students were discussing the assignment.
d) One of the boys are playing soccer.

Answer: b) Neither of the cats likes to play with toys. Explanation: In this sentence, "Neither" is a singular pronoun, so the verb "likes" should be singular as well, which is why it is the correct choice.

800. Which of the following sentences uses correct punctuation?
a) The doctor, said the nurse, was running late.
b) The doctor said the nurse, was running late.
c) The doctor, said the nurse was running late.
d) The doctor said the nurse was running late.

Answer: a) The doctor, said the nurse, was running late. Explanation: In this sentence, the phrase "said the nurse" is an interruption and should be set off by commas.

801. What is the main function of a predicate in a sentence?
a) To provide information about the subject
b) To introduce the main topic of the sentence
c) To express the action of the subject
d) To provide additional details about the topic

Answer: c) To express the action of the subject. Explanation: The predicate of a sentence is the part of the sentence that expresses the action or state of being of the subject.

802. Which of the following sentences is a compound sentence?
a) I like playing tennis, but I don't like playing football.
b) Although I like playing tennis, I am not very good at it.
c) I like playing tennis because it's a great workout.
d) I like playing tennis, it's a great workout.

Answer: a) I like playing tennis, but I don't like playing football. Explanation: A compound sentence contains two independent clauses joined by a coordinating conjunction. In this sentence, "I like playing tennis" and "I don't like playing football" are independent clauses joined by the conjunction "but".

803. Which of the following sentences is written in the passive voice?
a) The book was read by me.
b) I read the book.
c) The book is on the table.
d) The book has many pages.

Answer: a) The book was read by me. Explanation: In the passive voice, the subject of the sentence is acted upon by the verb. In this case, "the book" is the subject, and it is being acted upon by the verb "read".

804. Which of the following sentences correctly uses a semicolon?
a) I have a big test tomorrow; I can't go to the party.
b) I have a big test tomorrow, I can't go to the party.
c) I have a big test tomorrow: I can't go to the party.
d) I have a big test tomorrow - I can't go to the party.

Answer: a) I have a big test tomorrow; I can't go to the party. Explanation: A semicolon is used to join two closely related independent clauses in one sentence.

805. Which of the following sentences is a complex sentence?
a) I enjoy reading, and I like writing.
b) I enjoy reading, but I have no time because of work.
c) I enjoy reading because it is relaxing.
d) I enjoy reading; it is relaxing.

Answer: c) I enjoy reading because it is relaxing. Explanation: A complex sentence contains an independent clause and at least one dependent clause. In this sentence, "I enjoy reading" is the independent clause and "because it is relaxing" is the dependent clause.

806. Which type of sentence is used to express strong emotion or surprise?
a) Declarative sentence
b) Exclamatory sentence
c) Imperative sentence
d) Interrogative sentence

Answer: b) Exclamatory sentence. Explanation: Exclamatory sentences are used to express strong emotion or surprise. They often end with an exclamation mark.

807. Which of the following sentences correctly uses quotation marks?
a) My teacher said, "The test will be on Friday".
b) My teacher said "The test will be on Friday".
c) My teacher said "The test will be on Friday".
d) My teacher said, The test will be on Friday.

Answer: a) My teacher said, "The test will be on Friday". Explanation: Quotation marks should be used around direct quotes, and there should be a comma before the quote begins.

808. What is the purpose of an adverb in a sentence?
a) To describe a noun or pronoun
b) To express an action or state of being
c) To modify a verb, adjective, or other adverb
d) To show a relationship between two clauses

Answer: c) To modify a verb, adjective, or other adverb. Explanation: An adverb is a word that modifies a verb, an adjective, or another adverb. It can provide information about how, when, where, why, or to what extent something is done.

809. Which of the following sentences uses a colon correctly?
a) She has three favorite fruits: apples, oranges, and bananas.
b) She has: three favorite fruits apples, oranges, and bananas.
c) She has three favorite fruits: are apples, oranges, and bananas.
d) She has three favorite, fruits: apples, oranges, and bananas.

Answer: a) She has three favorite fruits: apples, oranges, and bananas. Explanation: A colon is used to introduce a list, a quote, or an explanation.

810. Which of the following sentences correctly uses an apostrophe?
a) The dogs' tails were wagging.
b) The dog's tail's were wagging.
c) The dogs tails' were wagging.
d) The dogs' tail's were wagging.

Answer: a) The dogs' tails were wagging. Explanation: The apostrophe is used to show possession. In this sentence, the tails belong to multiple dogs, so the apostrophe comes after the 's' in dogs.

811. Which of the following sentences uses a semicolon correctly?
a) She loves to read; she often reads before bed.
b) She loves to read, she often reads before bed;
c) She loves to read; because she often reads before bed.
d) She loves to read she often reads before bed;

Answer: a) She loves to read; she often reads before bed. Explanation: A semicolon is used to join two closely related independent clauses in one sentence.

812. Which punctuation mark is used to indicate a direct question?
a) Colon
b) Semicolon
c) Question mark
d) Exclamation point

Answer: c) Question mark. Explanation: A question mark is used at the end of a sentence to indicate a direct question.

813. What is the main function of a comma in a sentence?
a) To indicate the end of a sentence
b) To show excitement or emphasis
c) To separate items in a list
d) To indicate a direct question

Answer: c) To separate items in a list. Explanation: One of the main uses of a comma is to separate items in a list. Commas are also used to separate independent clauses when they are joined by a coordinating conjunction, and to set off introductory elements or interrupting elements in a sentence.

814. Which of the following sentences uses quotation marks correctly?
a) She said, "I'll see you tomorrow".
b) She said, "I'll see you tomorrow".
c) "She said, I'll see you tomorrow".
d) She said, I'll see you tomorrow.

Answer: b) She said, "I'll see you tomorrow". Explanation: Quotation marks are used to indicate direct speech. They should enclose the exact words that were spoken.

815. Which of the following sentences uses parentheses correctly?
a) She has two pets (a cat and a dog.
b) She has two pets a cat and a dog).
c) She has two pets (a cat and a dog).
d) She has two pets (a cat and a dog)

Answer: c) She has two pets (a cat and a dog). Explanation: Parentheses are used to add extra information or clarification in a sentence. The information inside the parentheses should be a complete thought or clarification of the information provided in the sentence.

816. What is the primary role of a period in written communication?
a) To indicate a pause or break
b) To show possession
c) To express strong emotion
d) To signal the end of a sentence

Answer: d) To signal the end of a sentence. Explanation: A period is used at the end of a sentence to indicate that the sentence is finished.

817. Which of the following sentences correctly uses a dash?
a) She has two hobbies--reading and writing.
b) She has--two hobbies reading and writing.
c) She has two hobbies--reading, and writing.
d) She has two hobbies reading and writing--.

Answer: a) She has two hobbies--reading and writing. Explanation: A dash is used to add extra information in a sentence, to show a range or connections, or to indicate an interruption. In this case, it is used to introduce a list.

818. Which punctuation mark is used to indicate surprise or strong emotion?
a) Colon
b) Semicolon
c) Exclamation point
d) Comma

Answer: c) Exclamation point. Explanation: An exclamation point is used at the end of a sentence to indicate surprise or strong emotion.

819. In the sentence "She was feeling quite melancholy," what does the word "melancholy" most likely mean?
a) Excited
b) Happy
c) Sad
d) Angry

Answer: c) Sad. Explanation: Context clues in the sentence suggest that "melancholy" is likely a negative emotion, and it often means a state of sadness or depression.

820. Which of the following strategies is not useful for understanding a difficult word in a text?
a) Looking at the surrounding context
b) Checking for prefixes or suffixes
c) Ignoring the word and hoping it's not important
d) Consulting a dictionary

Answer: c) Ignoring the word and hoping it's not important. Explanation: Ignoring the word won't help you understand it. Instead, use strategies like looking at context, examining word parts, or using a dictionary.

821. In the sentence "The robust man easily lifted the heavy boxes," what does the word "robust" most likely mean?
a) Weak
b) Sickly
c) Strong
d) Lazy

Answer: c) Strong. Explanation: The fact that the man "easily lifted the heavy boxes" provides a context clue that "robust" means strong.

822. What is the meaning of the prefix "un-" in the word "unhappy"?
a) Super
b) Not
c) Very
d) Over

Answer: b) Not. Explanation: The prefix "un-" negates the meaning of the word it's attached to. So, "unhappy" means "not happy."

823. In the sentence "She found the lecture to be tedious and long-winded," what does the word "tedious" most likely mean?
a) Exciting
b) Boring
c) Short
d) Thrilling

Answer: b) Boring. Explanation: The phrase "long-winded" provides a context clue that "tedious" likely means something negative, such as boring or uninteresting.

824. When you encounter an unfamiliar word while reading, what's the first strategy you should try?
a) Skip it
b) Look it up in a dictionary
c) Try to guess its meaning
d) Look at the context clues

Answer: d) Look at the context clues. Explanation: Using context clues provided by the sentence or paragraph often can give you a good idea of what the word means.

825. Which of the following is not a type of context clue?
a) Definition
b) Contrast
c) Punctuation
d) Inference

Answer: c) Punctuation. Explanation: Punctuation, while important for understanding sentence structure and tone, doesn't typically provide clues about the meaning of individual words.

826. In the sentence "His ludicrous suggestion made everyone laugh," what does the word "ludicrous" most likely mean?
a) Angry
b) Sad
c) Funny
d) Serious

Answer: c) Funny. Explanation: The fact that the suggestion "made everyone laugh" provides a context clue that "ludicrous" means funny or ridiculous.

827. What strategy can help you figure out the meaning of the word "unfriendly"?
a) Breaking the word into parts
b) Ignoring the word
c) Reading the sentence backwards
d) Changing the word order

Answer: a) Breaking the word into parts. Explanation: The word "unfriendly" can be broken into a prefix "un-", which means "not," and the base word "friendly." Thus, "unfriendly" means "not friendly."

828. In the sentence "The scenic view was breathtaking," what does the word "scenic" most likely mean?
a) Boring
b) Beautiful
c) Noisy
d) Unpleasant

Answer: b) Beautiful. Explanation: The word "breathtaking" provides a context clue that "scenic" is likely something positive and visually pleasing, like beautiful.

829. Which of the following words follows the 'i before e except after c' rule?
a) Siege
b) Ceiling
c) Science
d) Weird

Answer: b) Ceiling. Explanation: The word 'ceiling' follows the rule 'i before e, except after c'. In the word 'ceiling', 'e' comes before 'i' and it's after 'c'.

830. When adding a suffix beginning with a vowel to a word ending with a silent "e", what typically happens?
a) The silent "e" is dropped
b) The silent "e" is retained
c) The suffix is not added
d) The first letter of the word changes

Answer: a) The silent "e" is dropped. Explanation: Generally, when adding a suffix that begins with a vowel to a word ending in a silent "e", the "e" is dropped. For example, "hope" becomes "hoping", not "hopeing".

831. Which of the following words is spelled correctly?
a) Disappereance
b) Mischievous
c) Recieve
d) Sufferage

Answer: b) Mischievous. Explanation: "Mischievous" is spelled correctly according to standard English spelling conventions. The other options all have common spelling errors.

832. How does the spelling of a word ending in "y" typically change when adding a suffix?
a) The "y" is changed to "i"
b) The "y" is doubled
c) The "y" is dropped
d) The "y" is changed to "e"

Answer: a) The "y" is changed to "i". Explanation: In general, when adding a suffix to a word ending in "y", the "y" changes to "i". For example, "happy" becomes "happiness", not "happyness".

833. Which of the following is a correctly spelled plural form of a word ending in "f"?
a) Wolfs
b) Leafes
c) Loaves
d) Roofes

Answer: c) Loaves. Explanation: Some words ending in "f" change the "f" to "v" and add "es" to form the plural. "Loaf" becomes "loaves" in the plural.

834. Which of the following words is spelled correctly?
a) Priviledge
b) Accommadate
c) Embarrass
d) Calender

Answer: c) Embarrass. Explanation: "Embarrass" is spelled correctly according to standard English spelling conventions. The other options all have common spelling errors.

835. What typically happens to the final consonant in a one-syllable word when adding a suffix that begins with a vowel?
a) The consonant is doubled
b) The consonant is dropped
c) The consonant is changed to a vowel
d) The consonant remains the same

Answer: a) The consonant is doubled. Explanation: In most cases, when adding a suffix that starts with a vowel to a one-syllable word, the final consonant is doubled. For example, "run" becomes "running", not "runing".

836. Which of the following words is spelled correctly?
a) Accommodate
b) Exhilerate
c) Ocurence
d) Refference

Answer: a) Accommodate. Explanation: "Accommodate" is spelled correctly according to standard English spelling conventions. The other options all have common spelling errors.

837. Which spelling rule applies to the word "friendship"?
a) Change "y" to "i" when adding a suffix
b) Double the final consonant when adding a suffix
c) Drop the silent "e" when adding a suffix
d) No change when adding a suffix

Answer: d) No change when adding a suffix. Explanation: The word "friendship" adds the suffix "-ship" to "friend" without changing the original word, demonstrating the spelling rule that some words do not change when a suffix is added.

838. What is the plural form of the word "child"?
a) Childs
b) Children
c) Chilren
d) Childer

Answer: b) Children. Explanation: The word "child" is an irregular noun, and its plural form is "children", not "childs" or any other variation.

839. Why is it important for a nurse to be able to understand written medical instructions?
a) It allows the nurse to order supplies.
b) It enables the nurse to accurately administer patient care.
c) It is necessary for the nurse to pass board examinations.
d) It allows the nurse to communicate with insurance companies.

Answer: b) It enables the nurse to accurately administer patient care. Explanation: The ability to understand written medical instructions is crucial for a nurse to provide appropriate and accurate patient care. Misunderstanding instructions could lead to medical errors and compromised patient safety.

840. How does a nurse's comprehension of written medical research influence patient outcomes?
a) It helps the nurse to stay up-to-date with best practices.
b) It makes the nurse more competitive in the job market.
c) It enables the nurse to educate patients about their conditions.
d) Both a and c.

Answer: d) Both a and c. Explanation: By understanding medical research, a nurse can keep up with the latest best practices and provide high-quality care (option a), and also educate patients about their conditions to support informed decision-making (option c).

841. What role does written communication play in a nurse's collaboration with other healthcare professionals?
a) It ensures all parties have the same information.
b) It eliminates the need for verbal communication.
c) It allows the nurse to express personal opinions.
d) It creates a record of conversations.

Answer: a) It ensures all parties have the same information. Explanation: Written communication, such as in patient charts or via email, ensures that all healthcare professionals involved in a patient's care have access to the same information, supporting coordinated and effective care.

842. Which of the following is an example of how a nurse might use analytical reading skills in practice?
a) Writing a patient care report.
b) Reading a medication label.
c) Filling out an insurance form.
d) Documenting patient symptoms.

Answer: b) Reading a medication label. Explanation: Analytical reading skills are used to understand and interpret complex text, such as the information found on a medication label. This skill is crucial to ensure correct medication administration.

843. Why is it important for a nurse to be able to understand a patient's medical history as written in their medical record?
a) It allows the nurse to plan appropriate care for the patient.
b) It reduces the need for the nurse to interact with the patient.
c) It provides the nurse with information for billing purposes.
d) It allows the nurse to diagnose medical conditions.

Answer: a) It allows the nurse to plan appropriate care for the patient. Explanation: Understanding a patient's medical history as detailed in their record enables a nurse to plan and deliver care that is appropriate for the patient's specific needs and conditions.

844. How does the ability to comprehend written materials contribute to a nurse's effectiveness in patient education?
a) It reduces the amount of time the nurse needs to spend with each patient.
b) It enables the nurse to provide accurate information about health conditions and treatments.
c) It ensures the nurse can complete paperwork quickly.
d) It allows the nurse to understand and adhere to hospital policies.

Answer: b) It enables the nurse to provide accurate information about health conditions and treatments. Explanation: The ability to comprehend written materials, such as research studies or treatment guidelines, helps a nurse to provide accurate and helpful information to patients about their health conditions and treatments.

845. How does a nurse's ability to analyze written information affect patient safety?
a) It reduces the nurse's workload.
b) It ensures the nurse can understand and follow safety protocols.
c) It allows the nurse to communicate with non-English-speaking patients.
d) It enables the nurse to conduct medical research.

Answer: b) It ensures the nurse can understand and follow safety protocols. Explanation: The ability to analyze written information, such as safety protocols, is crucial for a nurse to ensure the safety of patients. If a nurse cannot understand or follow these guidelines, it could lead to mistakes that jeopardize patient safety.

846. Why is it important for a nurse to be able to understand written guidelines for patient care?
a) It allows the nurse to participate in hospital management.
b) It enables the nurse to provide care that is evidence-based and up-to-date.
c) It ensures the nurse can effectively communicate with patients.
d) It reduces the nurse's reliance on coworkers for information.

Answer: b) It enables the nurse to provide care that is evidence-based and up-to-date. Explanation: Written guidelines for patient care often reflect the latest evidence-based best practices. A nurse who can understand these guidelines can provide care that is up-to-date and effective.

847. Why might a nurse need to be able to understand written materials outside their specific area of expertise?
a) It enables the nurse to provide holistic care.
b) It allows the nurse to manage the hospital.
c) It ensures the nurse can work in any department.
d) It reduces the need for the nurse to seek help from others.

Answer: a) It enables the nurse to provide holistic care. Explanation: Healthcare is interdisciplinary, and a patient's health can be affected by a wide range of factors. By being able to understand written materials across different healthcare disciplines, a nurse can provide holistic care that takes into account all aspects of a patient's health.

848. How might a nurse's ability to understand written patient feedback contribute to the quality of care?
a) It allows the nurse to respond to patient complaints.
b) It enables the nurse to adjust care based on patient feedback.
c) It ensures the nurse can defend themselves against criticism.
d) It provides the nurse with a sense of job satisfaction.

Answer: b) It enables the nurse to adjust care based on patient feedback. Explanation: Understanding written patient feedback can give a nurse valuable insights into how care could be improved. By adjusting care in response to this feedback, the nurse can help to enhance the quality of care provided.

849. Which of the following sentences correctly uses the word "complement"?
a) She received a nice complement on her new outfit.
b) The moon complements the stars in the night sky.
c) I would like a side complement with my dinner.
d) The dancers made a complement to the music with their movements.

Answer: b) The moon complements the stars in the night sky. Explanation: "Complement" refers to something that completes or goes well with something. In this sentence, the moon is said to complement the stars, meaning it enhances the beauty or completeness of the night sky.

850. Which of the following words is spelled correctly?
a) Recieve
b) Procede
c) Perceive
d) Decieve

Answer: c) Perceive. Explanation: The correct spelling of the words should be "receive," "proceed," and "deceive," following the rule "i before e except after c."

851. The word 'elicit' is used correctly in which of the following sentences?
a) He tried to elicit the correct answer from his memory.
b) The artist elicits paintings with vibrant colors.
c) She tried to elicit her family history in her book.
d) The teacher was known for his ability to elicit attention.

Answer: a) He tried to elicit the correct answer from his memory. Explanation: The word 'elicit' means to draw out or provoke. In this context, the person is trying to draw out the correct answer from his memory.

852. Choose the sentence where the word 'principal' is used correctly.
a) The principal reason for my visit is to see the Eiffel Tower.
b) The principle of the matter is that he lied.
c) The principal of the recipe is flour.
d) He held onto his principles and refused to lie.

Answer: a) The principal reason for my visit is to see the Eiffel Tower. Explanation: 'Principal' as an adjective means main or most important. In this sentence, it is used correctly to indicate that the main reason for the visit is to see the Eiffel Tower.

853. Which sentence uses correct punctuation?
a) The dog, chased its tail.
b) The dog chased its, tail.
c) The dog chased its tail.
d) The, dog chased its tail.

Answer: c) The dog chased its tail. Explanation: There is no need for commas in this simple sentence. The subject is 'the dog' and the predicate is 'chased its tail'.

854. Which of the following words is an example of a homophone?
a) Bear
b) Rare
c) Pair
d) Stare

Answer: c) Pair. Explanation: A homophone is a word that is pronounced the same as another word but differs in meaning. 'Pair' is a homophone of 'pear'.

855. Which sentence is grammatically correct?
a) Their going to the mall later.
b) They're going to the mall later.
c) There going to the mall later.
d) Thier going to the mall later.

Answer: b) They're going to the mall later. Explanation: 'They're' is the contraction of 'they are', and it is used correctly in this sentence. The other options misuse homophones of 'they're'.

856. What does the prefix 'sub-' mean in the word 'submerge'?
a) Above
b) Under
c) Around
d) Between

Answer: b) Under. Explanation: In the word 'submerge', the prefix 'sub-' means 'under'. Therefore, 'submerge' means to go under water.

857. Which of the following demonstrates correct use of the word 'affect'?
a) The affect of the music was soothing.
b) She had a happy affect.
c) The rain did not affect their plans.
d) The affect was immediate and startling.

Answer: c) The rain did not affect their plans. Explanation: 'Affect' is most commonly used as a verb meaning to influence. In this sentence, it's used correctly to indicate that the rain didn't influence or change their plans.

858. Which of the following words is spelled correctly?
a) Accomodate
b) Believe
c) Recieve
d) Definately

Answer: b) Believe. Explanation: The word "believe" follows the standard rule of "i before e except after c."

859. She baked the _____ to perfection. Which of the following options correctly completes the sentence above?
a) Coffee
b) Cake
c) Table
d) Chair

Answer: b) Cake. Explanation: The verb "baked" in the sentence indicates that the blank must be filled with something that can be baked, which is "cake" in this case.

860. My _____ has many tips on finding deals at the grocery store. Which of the following options correctly completes the sentence above?
a) Sneaker
b) Lamp
c) Book
d) Sunglasses

Answer: c) Book. Explanation: The context of the sentence suggests that the blank must be filled with something that can contain tips or advice. In this case, "book" is the best fit.

861. Which of the following sentences shows the correct use of punctuation marks?
a) I love cooking, my dog, and reading.
b) I love cooking my dog and reading.
c) I love cooking, my dog and reading.
d) I love cooking my dog, and reading.

Answer: a) I love cooking, my dog, and reading. Explanation: This sentence uses the Oxford comma correctly to separate three distinct items or activities.

862. To prepare the entree, the chef mixed olive oil, chicken, and vegetables. Which of the following correctly punctuates the sentence above?
a) To prepare the entree the chef mixed olive oil chicken and vegetables.
b) To prepare the entree, the chef mixed: olive oil, chicken, and vegetables.
c) To prepare the entree, the chef mixed olive oil chicken and vegetables.
d) To prepare the entree, the chef mixed olive oil chicken, and vegetables.

Answer: c) To prepare the entree, the chef mixed olive oil, chicken, and vegetables. Explanation: This sentence correctly uses commas to separate items in a list.

863. Our mail carrier _____. Which of the following predicates correctly completes the sentence above?
a) Across the street
b) Every morning
c) Delivers mail
d) Blue uniform

Answer: c) Delivers mail. Explanation: This predicate completes the sentence by providing an action for the subject 'our mail carrier'.

864. Which of the following would most likely act as a transition sentence?
a) "However, not all scientists agree on this point."
b) "The sun is a star."
c) "The moon orbits the Earth."
d) "Some planets have moons."

Answer: a) "However, not all scientists agree on this point." Explanation: This sentence introduces a contrast or shift in perspective, which is a common function of transition sentences.

865. Which of the following sentences would most likely act as a supporting detail?
a) "Climate change is a significant issue."
b) "According to the Environmental Protection Agency, global temperatures have risen by 1.9 degrees Fahrenheit since 1880."
c) "There are many causes of climate change."
d) "We must take action to mitigate the effects of climate change."

Answer: b) "According to the Environmental Protection Agency, global temperatures have risen by 1.9 degrees Fahrenheit since 1880." Explanation: This sentence provides specific data to support a broader statement or argument, which is typical of a supporting detail.

866. In order to run a successful business, you have to prioritize your company's overall performance rather than relying solely on a few customer reviews. Which of the following words are spelled incorrectly in the sentence above? Select all that apply.
a) Buisness
b) Prioritize
c) Performance
d) Soley

Answer: a) Buisness, d) Soley. Explanation: The correct spellings are "business" and "solely".

867. Which of the following sentences correctly uses the verb "lie"?
a) I will lay down for a nap.
b) I will lie down for a nap.
c) I will laid down for a nap.
d) I will lied down for a nap.

Answer: b) I will lie down for a nap. Explanation: "Lie" is an intransitive verb that means to recline, and it does not require a direct object.

868. Which of the following sentences correctly uses punctuation?
a) The books are on the table; the pencils, on the shelf.
b) The books are on the table the pencils on the shelf.
c) The books, are on the table; the pencils, on the shelf.
d) The books are on the table; the pencils on the shelf, .

Answer: a) The books are on the table; the pencils, on the shelf. Explanation: This sentence correctly uses a semicolon to separate related independent clauses and a comma for apposition.

869. Which word best fills in the blank in the following sentence? "The lecturer had a very _____ voice that put most of the audience to sleep."
a) Monotonous
b) Monogamous
c) Monolithic
d) Monotonic

Answer: a) Monotonous. Explanation: The context of the sentence suggests that the lecturer's voice was unvarying in tone, which is what "monotonous" means.

870. Which sentence correctly uses the word "principal"?
a) The principle of the school is strict.
b) The principal reason I am late is because of traffic.
c) I have a principal in my back.
d) I have a lot of principals.

Answer: b) The principal reason I am late is because of traffic. Explanation: "Principal" can mean main or most important, which is the correct usage in option b.

871. Which of the following sentences correctly uses the homophones "their," "they're," and "there"?
a) There going to their house over there.
b) Their going to they're house over there.
c) They're going to their house over there.
d) Their going to their house over there.

Answer: c) They're going to their house over there. Explanation: This sentence correctly uses "they're" (a contraction of "they are"), "their" (possessive form of "they"), and "there" (a place).

872. Which of the following sentences has an incorrect modifier?
a) The dog that barks loudly is mine.
b) The man with the tall hat waved.
c) I found a golden man's watch.
d) Running fast, the scenery passed in a blur.

Answer: c) I found a golden man's watch. Explanation: This sentence incorrectly implies that the man is golden rather than the watch. The correct phrasing is "I found a man's golden watch."

873. Which of the following sentences has the correct subject-verb agreement?
a) The staff at the hospital is very friendly.
b) The staff at the hospital are very friendly.
c) The bunch of grapes are ripe.
d) A group of musicians are playing.

Answer: a) The staff at the hospital is very friendly. Explanation: When "staff" is used to mean a group of people as a single entity, it takes a singular verb.

874. Which of the following sentences has a misplaced modifier?
a) Having finished the assignment, the Xbox was my next target.
b) I ate only the apples in the bowl.
c) The hikers saw a mountain in the distance covered in snow.
d) The teacher handed out the textbooks that were brand new.

Answer: a) Having finished the assignment, the Xbox was my next target. Explanation: The modifier "having finished the assignment" is misplaced because it is closer to "the Xbox" and makes the sentence seem as though the Xbox finished the assignment. A correct version would be "Having finished the assignment, I targeted the Xbox next."

875. Which of the following sentences has correct pronoun-antecedent agreement?
a) Every student should do their homework.
b) Neither of the boys brought their umbrella.
c) Each of the girls did her job.
d) Somebody has left its umbrella.

Answer: c) Each of the girls did her job. Explanation: The antecedent "each" is singular, so it should have a singular pronoun like "her".

876. Which of the following sentences correctly uses an adverb?
a) He drives safe.
b) She sings beautifully.
c) He feels badly about forgetting her birthday.
d) I feel strongly about this issue.

Answer: b) She sings beautifully. Explanation: The adverb "beautifully" correctly modifies the verb "sings" to describe how the singing is done.

877. Which of the following sentences demonstrates the correct use of commas in a list?
a) I need to buy milk, bread and, eggs at the grocery store.
b) I need to buy milk, bread, eggs at the grocery store.
c) I need to buy milk, bread, and eggs at the grocery store.
d) I need to buy, milk, bread, and eggs at the grocery store.

Answer: c) I need to buy milk, bread, and eggs at the grocery store. Explanation: Commas are used to separate items in a list and should be placed after each item except the last one, where 'and' is used.

878. Which of the following sentences correctly uses the conjunction "so"?
a) I didn't study for the test so I failed.
b) I didn't study for the test, so I failed.
c) I didn't study for the test so, I failed.
d) I didn't, study for the test so I failed.

Answer: b) I didn't study for the test, so I failed. Explanation: The conjunction "so" connects two independent clauses and a comma is usually used before it.

879. Which of the following is a correctly spelled word?
a) Accomodate
b) Misspell
c) Recieve
d) Seperate

Answer: b) Misspell. Explanation: This is the only option that is spelled correctly. The others are common misspellings.

880. Which sentence correctly uses a semicolon?
a) The cake is sweet; it is also very moist.
b) The cake is sweet, it is also very moist.
c) The cake is sweet; and it is also very moist.
d) The cake is sweet it is also very moist.

Answer: a) The cake is sweet; it is also very moist. Explanation: A semicolon can be used to connect closely related independent clauses.

881. Which of the following sentences correctly uses an apostrophe?
a) The cats' tail is long.
b) The cat's tail's are long.
c) The cat's tails is long.
d) The cats tail's are long.

Answer: a) The cats' tail is long. Explanation: An apostrophe is used to indicate possession. "Cats'" indicates that the tail belongs to one cat.

882. Which of the following sentences correctly uses "fewer" and "less"?
a) There are less apples in the basket than oranges.
b) I have fewer money than I did yesterday.
c) She has less books than me.
d) There are fewer chairs here than before.

Answer: d) There are fewer chairs here than before. Explanation: "Fewer" is used with countable nouns, while "less" is used with uncountable nouns.

883. Which of the following sentences has a correctly placed modifier?
a) The man walking the dogs in the park is my uncle.
b) The man in the park walking the dogs is my uncle.
c) The man is my uncle in the park walking the dogs.
d) The man walking in the park the dogs is my uncle.

Answer: a) The man walking the dogs in the park is my uncle. Explanation: The phrase "walking the dogs in the park" correctly modifies "the man".

884. Which of the following sentences uses correct subject-verb agreement?
a) The pair of shoes I bought are too small.
b) The pair of shoes I bought is too small.
c) The pair of shoes I bought were too small.
d) The pair of shoes I bought have been too small.

Answer: b) The pair of shoes I bought is too small. Explanation: When "pair" is the subject, it takes a singular verb, as it refers to one pair.

885. Which sentence correctly uses a reflexive pronoun?
a) I myself baked these cookies.
b) Himself likes to run in the mornings.
c) They went to the park themselves.
d) I gave herself a gift.

Answer: a) I myself baked these cookies. Explanation: Reflexive pronouns are used for emphasis or to indicate that the subject of the verb is also its object.

886. Which of the following sentences uses "me" and "I" correctly?
a) My friend and me went to the park.
b) My friend and I went to the park.
c) Me and my friend went to the park.
d) The park was visited by my friend and I.

Answer: b) My friend and I went to the park. Explanation: When used as a subject, "I" is the correct pronoun to use.

887. Which sentence correctly uses a hyphen?
a) My grandmother is eighty-five years old.
b) My grandmother is eighty five years old.
c) My grandmother is eighty five-years old.
d) My grandmother is eighty-five-years old.

Answer: a) My grandmother is eighty-five years old. Explanation: A hyphen is used to connect words that function together as an adjective, like "eighty-five".

888. In the following sentence, which word is an example of a homophone? "She went to the beach to see the sea."
a) Went
b) Beach
c) See
d) Sea

Answer: c) See and d) Sea. Explanation: Homophones are words that are pronounced the same but have different meanings. "See" and "Sea" are homophones.

889. Which of the following sentences correctly uses the word "there", "their", or "they're"?
a) There going to the movies tonight.
b) Their is no milk left in the fridge.
c) They're dog is very friendly.
d) They're going to the movies tonight.

Answer: d) They're going to the movies tonight. Explanation: "They're" is a contraction of "they are".

890. Which of the following words is an antonym of "joyful"?
a) Happy
b) Excited
c) Gleeful
d) Miserable

Answer: d) Miserable. Explanation: An antonym is a word that has the opposite meaning. "Miserable" is the opposite of "joyful".

891. Which of the following sentences demonstrates correct use of a colon?
a) I bought three things at the store: milk, bread and eggs.
b) I bought three things at the store, milk: bread and eggs.
c) I bought three things at the store, milk, bread: and eggs.
d) I bought three things: at the store: milk, bread, and eggs.

Answer: a) I bought three things at the store: milk, bread and eggs. Explanation: A colon is used before a list or an explanation that is preceded by a clause that can stand by itself.

892. Which of the following sentences correctly uses "who" and "whom"?
a) Whom is going to the store?
b) I don't know who to give this to.
c) To who should I address this letter?
d) Whom should I say is calling?

Answer: d) Whom should I say is calling? Explanation: "Whom" is used as the object of a verb or preposition.

893. Which of the following words is a synonym for "fast"?
a) Slow
b) Rapid
c) Delayed
d) Lengthy

Answer: b) Rapid. Explanation: A synonym is a word that has the same or similar meaning. "Rapid" is a synonym for "fast".

894. Which sentence correctly uses a contraction?
a) Your going to love this movie.
b) You're book is on the table.
c) You're going to love this movie.
d) Your going to the store later.

Answer: c) You're going to love this movie. Explanation: "You're" is a contraction of "you are".

895. Which sentence correctly uses "its" and "it's"?
a) Its raining outside.
b) The dog wagged it's tail.
c) It's tail is very fluffy.
d) It's raining outside.

Answer: d) It's raining outside. Explanation: "It's" is a contraction of "it is" or "it has". "Its" is a possessive pronoun.

896. Which of the following sentences demonstrates the correct use of a comma in a direct address?
a) "I'm telling you Sarah, it's not worth it."
b) "I'm telling you, Sarah it's not worth it."
c) "I'm telling you, Sarah, it's not worth it."
d) "I'm telling, you Sarah it's not worth it."

Answer: c) "I'm telling you, Sarah, it's not worth it." Explanation: Commas are used to separate the name of the person being addressed from the rest of the sentence.

897. Which of the following words correctly completes the sentence: "I _____ to the store to buy some groceries."
a) went
b) goed
c) go
d) goes

Answer: a) went. Explanation: In this context, the past tense of "go" is required, which is "went".

898. Which of the following sentences is grammatically correct?
a) Me and my friend likes to play basketball.
b) I and my friend likes to play basketball.
c) My friend and I likes to play basketball.
d) My friend and I like to play basketball.

Answer: d) My friend and I like to play basketball. Explanation: When combining subjects, the pronoun "I" should be last. Also, the verb should agree with the plural subject "my friend and I".

899. In the following sentence, which punctuation is incorrect? "She asked, "Can I borrow a pencil?"
a) The comma
b) The first quotation mark
c) The second quotation mark
d) The question mark

Answer: c) The second quotation mark. Explanation: In American English, punctuation marks are placed inside the quotation marks. So it should be: "She asked, "Can I borrow a pencil?"

900. Which word correctly completes the sentence: "He _____ a book about ancient civilizations."
a) written
b) wrote
c) writed
d) write

Answer: b) wrote. Explanation: The past tense of "write" is "wrote", which is needed in this context.

901. Which of the following is an example of a compound sentence?
a) I like apples.
b) I like apples, but I do not like oranges.
c) I do not like oranges.
d) Apples are my favorite fruit.

Answer: b) I like apples, but I do not like oranges. Explanation: A compound sentence contains two independent clauses joined by a coordinating conjunction (for, and, nor, but, or, yet, so).

902. Which of the following sentences uses an apostrophe correctly?
a) The dogs' are in the yard.
b) The dog's are in the yard.
c) The dogs bone is in the yard.
d) The dog's bone is in the yard.

Answer: d) The dog's bone is in the yard. Explanation: The apostrophe in "dog's" indicates possession.

903. Which of the following sentences contains an adverb?
a) She runs quickly.
b) She runs in the park.
c) She runs every day.
d) She runs fastly.

Answer: a) She runs quickly. Explanation: An adverb is a word that modifies a verb, an adjective, or another adverb. "Quickly" is an adverb in this sentence.

904. Which of the following sentences demonstrates the correct usage of the words "your" and "you're"?
a) Your going to the store later.
b) You're book is over there.
c) You're going to the store later.
d) Your going to love this book.

Answer: c) You're going to the store later. Explanation: "You're" is a contraction of "you are". "Your" is a possessive pronoun.

905. Which of the following sentences is written in the passive voice?
a) The dog chased the cat.
b) The cat was chased by the dog.
c) The cat chased the dog.
d) The dog was chased by the cat.

Answer: b) The cat was chased by the dog. Explanation: In the passive voice, the subject receives the action of the verb.

906. Which of the following words correctly completes the sentence: "I _____ like to study in the library."
a) doesn't
b) don't
c) isn't
d) aren't

Answer: b) don't. Explanation: "I don't" is the correct contraction of "I do not". The other choices are incorrect in this context.

907. In which sentence is the semicolon used correctly?
a) I have a big test tomorrow; I can't go to the concert.
b) I have a big test; tomorrow, I can't go to the concert.
c) I have a big test tomorrow I can't; go to the concert.
d) I have a big test tomorrow; and I can't go to the concert.

Answer: a) I have a big test tomorrow; I can't go to the concert. Explanation: A semicolon is used to join two related independent clauses.

908. Which of the following sentences uses correct subject-verb agreement?
a) The students enjoys the class.
b) The student enjoy the class.
c) The students enjoy the class.
d) The student enjoys the class.

Answer: d) The student enjoys the class. Explanation: The singular subject "student" requires the singular verb form "enjoys".

909. Which of the following sentences correctly uses the pronoun "its"?
a) Its raining outside.
b) The dog wagged it's tail.
c) The dog wagged its tail.
d) It's color is blue.

Answer: c) The dog wagged its tail. Explanation: "Its" is a possessive pronoun.

910. Which of the following sentences is an example of a complex sentence?
a) I love reading, and I enjoy writing.
b) I love reading.
c) I love reading because it's relaxing.
d) I love reading, but I also enjoy writing.

Answer: c) I love reading because it's relaxing. Explanation: A complex sentence contains an independent clause and at least one dependent clause.

911. Which of the following sentences is punctuated correctly?
a) "Where are you going?" asked John.
b) "Where are you going asked John."
c) "Where are you going?" Asked John.
d) "Where are you going" asked John.

Answer: a) "Where are you going?" asked John. Explanation: In dialogue, a question mark is used at the end of a direct question and it goes inside the quotation marks.

912. What is the correct plural form of the noun "thesis"?
a) thesises
b) thesis
c) thesiss
d) theses

Answer: d) theses. Explanation: The plural form of "thesis" is "theses".

913. Which sentence correctly uses the word "whose"?
a) I don't know whose going to the party.
b) Whose is that book?
c) Whose book is that?
d) I don't know, whose going?

Answer: c) Whose book is that? Explanation: "Whose" is a possessive pronoun used to indicate ownership.

914. Which of the following words correctly completes the sentence: "If I _____ you, I would study more."
a) was
b) were
c) am
d) be

Answer: b) were. Explanation: The subjunctive mood is used for hypothetical situations and requires the base form of the verb, "were", even with singular subjects.

915. Which of the following sentences is an example of a declarative sentence?
a) Is that your book?
b) Please pass the salt.
c) I enjoy reading.
d) Stop!

Answer: c) I enjoy reading. Explanation: A declarative sentence makes a statement or expresses an opinion.

916. Which of the following sentences demonstrates the correct usage of a comma?
a) I need to buy milk eggs and bread.
b) I need to buy milk, eggs and bread.
c) I need to buy milk eggs, and bread.
d) I need, to buy milk, eggs and bread.

Answer: b) I need to buy milk, eggs and bread. Explanation: In a list, commas are used to separate items. This is known as a serial comma or Oxford comma.

917. Which of the following sentences uses the correct form of "there/their/they're"?
a) Their going to the movies later.
b) There going to the movies later.
c) They're going to the movies later.
d) The're going to the movies later.

Answer: c) They're going to the movies later. Explanation: "They're" is a contraction of "they are".

918. Which sentence correctly uses the phrase "in regard to"?
a) I have some concerns in regards to your proposal.
b) I have some concerns in regard to your proposal.
c) In regard to your proposal, I have some concerns.
d) Both b and c

Answer: d) Both b and c. Explanation: The correct phrase is "in regard to".

919. Which sentence demonstrates correct usage of the colon?
a) Here's what I need: milk, eggs, and bread.
b) Here's what I need, milk: eggs, and bread.
c) Here's what I need: milk, eggs and, bread.
d) Here's what I need milk: eggs, and bread.

Answer: a) Here's what I need: milk, eggs, and bread. Explanation: A colon is used to introduce a list or a definition.

920. What is the correct past tense of the verb "go"?
a) goed
b) gone
c) went
d) go

Answer: c) went. Explanation: The past tense of "go" is "went".

921. Which sentence correctly uses the word "its"?
a) Its raining outside.
b) The cat is licking it's paw.
c) The cat is licking its paw.
d) The book lost it's cover.

Answer: c) The cat is licking its paw. Explanation: "Its" is a possessive pronoun.

922. Which of the following sentences is an example of an interrogative sentence?
a) Do you know what time it is?
b) I can't believe it's already noon.
c) Make sure to finish your homework.
d) It's a beautiful day outside.

Answer: a) Do you know what time it is? Explanation: An interrogative sentence asks a question.

923. What is the correct comparative form of the adjective "good"?
a) gooder
b) more good
c) better
d) best

Answer: c) better. Explanation: The comparative form of "good" is "better".

924. Which of the following sentences is an example of a compound sentence?
a) I love reading.
b) I love reading, and I enjoy writing.
c) I love reading because it's relaxing.
d) I love reading, but I also enjoy writing.

Answer: b) I love reading, and I enjoy writing. Explanation: A compound sentence contains two or more independent clauses joined by a coordinating conjunction.

925. Which of the following sentences is punctuated correctly?
a) "Where are you going asked John."
b) "Where are you going," asked John.
c) "Where are you going"? asked John.
d) "Where are you going?" asked John.

Answer: d) "Where are you going?" asked John. Explanation: In dialogue, a question mark is used at the end of a direct question and it goes inside the quotation marks.

926. Which sentence correctly uses the word "who's"?
a) Who's book is this?
b) Who's going to the party?
c) I don't know who's car this is.
d) This is the man who's dog was lost.

Answer: b) Who's going to the party? Explanation: "Who's" is a contraction of "who is" or "who has".

927. Choose the sentence that correctly uses a semicolon.
a) I have a big test tomorrow; I can't go to the concert.
b) I have a big test tomorrow, I can't go to the concert.
c) I have a big test tomorrow; and I can't go to the concert.
d) I have a big test tomorrow; because I can't go to the concert.

Answer: a) I have a big test tomorrow; I can't go to the concert. Explanation: Semicolons are used to connect two related independent clauses.

928. Which of the following sentences uses the correct form of "your/you're"?
a) Your late for class.
b) You're backpack is in the car.
c) Your the best teacher I've ever had.
d) You're going to love this movie.

Answer: d) You're going to love this movie. Explanation: "You're" is a contraction of "you are".

929. Choose the sentence that is punctuated correctly.
a) My favorite books are: Harry Potter, Lord of the Rings, and Pride and Prejudice.
b) My favorite books are Harry Potter, Lord of the Rings, and Pride and Prejudice.
c) My favorite books are: Harry Potter, Lord of the Rings and Pride and Prejudice.
d) My favorite books are, Harry Potter, Lord of the Rings, and Pride and Prejudice.

Answer: b) My favorite books are Harry Potter, Lord of the Rings, and Pride and Prejudice. Explanation: In a list, a colon should not be used after a verb or preposition.

930. What is the correct past participle of the verb "write"?
a) writed
b) wrote
c) written
d) writen

Answer: c) written. Explanation: The past participle of "write" is "written".

931. Which sentence correctly uses the word "its"?
a) Its cold outside.
b) Its time to go home.
c) The dog wagged its tail.
d) I can't find my phone, its missing.

Answer: c) The dog wagged its tail. Explanation: "Its" is a possessive pronoun.

932. Which of the following sentences is an example of a declarative sentence?
a) Will you help me with my homework?
b) Help me with my homework.
c) My homework is very difficult.
d) What a difficult homework assignment!

Answer: c) My homework is very difficult. Explanation: A declarative sentence makes a statement or provides information.

933. What is the correct superlative form of the adjective "bad"?
a) badder
b) more bad
c) baddest
d) worst

Answer: d) worst. Explanation: The superlative form of "bad" is "worst".

934. Which of the following sentences is an example of a complex sentence?
a) I love reading.
b) I love reading, and I enjoy writing.
c) I love reading because it's relaxing.
d) I love reading, but I also enjoy writing.

Answer: c) I love reading because it's relaxing. Explanation: A complex sentence contains one independent clause and at least one dependent clause.

935. Which of the following sentences is punctuated correctly?
a) "How are you" John asked.
b) "How are you," John asked.
c) "How are you"? John asked.
d) "How are you?" John asked.

Answer: d) "How are you?" John asked. Explanation: In dialogue, a question mark is used at the end of a direct question and it goes inside the quotation marks.

936. Which sentence correctly uses the word "whose"?
a) Whose going to the party?
b) I don't know whose going.
c) Whose book is this?
d) This is the man whose going to the party.

Answer: c) Whose book is this? Explanation: "Whose" is a possessive pronoun.

937. Which sentence is correctly written in the active voice?
a) The cookies were baked by my grandmother.
b) My homework was finished before dinner.
c) The cat was chased by the dog.
d) The teacher graded the tests quickly.

Answer: d) The teacher graded the tests quickly. Explanation: Active voice occurs when the subject of the sentence is performing the action.

938. Choose the correct verb to fill in the blank: The group of students __ at the library every Tuesday.
a) meet
b) meets
c) meeting
d) met

Answer: b) meets. Explanation: When the subject of a sentence is a collective noun referring to a group as a single entity, a singular verb is used.

939. Which sentence correctly uses a plural possessive noun?
a) The childrens toys were scattered all over the floor.
b) The children's toys were scattered all over the floor.
c) The childrens' toys were scattered all over the floor.
d) The children toy's were scattered all over the floor.

Answer: b) The children's toys were scattered all over the floor. Explanation: When making a plural noun that does not end in "s" possessive, you add an apostrophe and "s".

940. Which sentence is an example of a compound-complex sentence?
a) I like to read, and I enjoy jogging.
b) I like to read, and I enjoy jogging because it's refreshing.
c) I like to read because it's fun.
d) Because I like to read, I have many books.

Answer: b) I like to read, and I enjoy jogging because it's refreshing. Explanation: A compound-complex sentence consists of at least two independent clauses and one or more dependent clauses.

941. Which word is a synonym for "beautiful"?
a) Ugly
b) Plain
c) Stunning
d) Simple

Answer: c) Stunning. Explanation: Synonyms are words that have similar meanings.

942. Choose the correct spelling of the word:
a) Recieve
b) Recive
c) Receive
d) Receve

Answer: c) Receive. Explanation: The correct spelling is "receive". Remember, "i" before "e" except after "c".

943. Which sentence is an example of an exclamatory sentence?
a) Can you help me with this?
b) Please help me with this.
c) I need help with this.
d) What a beautiful sunset!

Answer: d) What a beautiful sunset! Explanation: Exclamatory sentences express strong emotion and end with an exclamation point.

944. What is the correct plural form of "mouse"?
a) Mouses
b) Mouse's
c) Mice
d) Mouse

Answer: c) Mice. Explanation: The plural form of "mouse" is "mice".

945. Which sentence correctly uses the word "there"?
a) There books are on the table.
b) They're going to the park.
c) Their is no reason to be upset.
d) There is a great movie playing tonight.

Answer: d) There is a great movie playing tonight. Explanation: "There" is used to refer to a place, or to indicate the existence of something.

946. Which sentence correctly uses the word "then"?
a) I am taller then you.
b) We went to the park, and then we went to the movies.
c) I would rather eat pizza then pasta.
d) I have more then enough time.

Answer: b) We went to the park, and then we went to the movies. Explanation: "Then" is used to indicate a sequence in time or a consequence.

947. In which sentence is the verb in the present perfect tense?
a) I eat breakfast every morning.
b) I have eaten breakfast already.
c) I was eating breakfast when you called.
d) I will eat breakfast after I finish this.

Answer: b) I have eaten breakfast already. Explanation: The present perfect tense is formed with "have/has" + past participle.

948. Which sentence is written in the passive voice?
a) The tree was hit by the car.
b) The car hit the tree.
c) The tree hits the car.
d) The tree is hitting the car.

Answer: a) The tree was hit by the car. Explanation: In the passive voice, the subject receives the action.

949. Which word is the correct relative pronoun to complete this sentence: The man __ car broke down is waiting for a tow truck.
a) whose
b) who's
c) whos
d) who

Answer: a) whose. Explanation: "Whose" is a relative pronoun used to indicate possession.

950. What is the correct plural form of the word "cactus"?
a) Cactuses
b) Cactus's
c) Cacti
d) Cactus

Answer: c) Cacti. Explanation: Some nouns ending in "us" from Latin origin have their plural formed by changing "us" to "i".

951. Which sentence correctly uses an apostrophe to show possession?
a) The dogs tail is wagging.
b) The dogs' tail is wagging.
c) The dog's tail is wagging.
d) The dog tail's is wagging.

Answer: c) The dog's tail is wagging. Explanation: An apostrophe is used before the "s" to show singular possession.

952. Which sentence correctly uses a coordinating conjunction?
a) I like to run, but I don't like to swim.
b) I like to run but, I don't like to swim.
c) I like to run, but, I don't like to swim.
d) I like to run but I don't like to swim.

Answer: a) I like to run, but I don't like to swim. Explanation: Coordinating conjunctions (for, and, nor, but, or, yet, so) connect words, phrases, and clauses.

953. Which word correctly fills in the blank in this sentence: He acted as though he ___ seen a ghost.
a) had
b) has
c) have
d) having

Answer: a) had. Explanation: The past perfect tense (had + past participle) is used in this hypothetical past situation.

954. Which sentence correctly uses a semicolon?
a) I have a big test tomorrow; I can't go to the concert.
b) I have a big test tomorrow, I can't go to the concert.
c) I have a big test tomorrow,; I can't go to the concert.
d) I have a big test tomorrow I can't go to the concert.

Answer: a) I have a big test tomorrow; I can't go to the concert. Explanation: A semicolon is used to link two independent clauses that are closely related in thought.

955. Which word correctly fills in the blank in this sentence: I was ___ tired that I fell asleep as soon as I got home.
a) to
b) too
c) two
d) tu

Answer: b) too. Explanation: "Too" is an adverb that can mean "excessively" or "also".

956. Which sentence correctly uses quotation marks?
a) My mom said, get your shoes on.
b) My mom said "get your shoes on."
c) My mom said, "Get your shoes on."
d) My mom said "Get your shoes on".

Answer: c) My mom said, "Get your shoes on." Explanation: Quotation marks are used to show the exact words someone said, and they are placed after the comma that follows the dialogue tag.

957. What is the correct past tense form of the irregular verb "run"?
a) Runned
b) Run
c) Ran
d) Running

Answer: c) Ran. Explanation: The past tense form of "run" is "ran."

958. Which of the following words is an example of an adverb?
a) Quick
b) Quickly
c) Quicken
d) Quickest

Answer: b) Quickly. Explanation: Adverbs often end in "-ly" and describe or modify verbs.

959. What is the correct comparative form of the adjective "bad"?
a) Badder
b) Badest
c) Worse
d) Worst

Answer: c) Worse. Explanation: The comparative form of "bad" is "worse."

960. What type of sentence is this: "Close the door."
a) Declarative
b) Interrogative
c) Exclamatory
d) Imperative

Answer: d) Imperative. Explanation: Imperative sentences give commands or make requests.

961. Which sentence is written in the active voice?
a) The ball was thrown by John.
b) John was thrown by the ball.
c) John threw the ball.
d) The ball is being thrown by John.

Answer: c) John threw the ball. Explanation: In active voice, the subject performs the action.

962. Which of the following sentences is an example of correct subject-verb agreement?
a) The team are winning the game.
b) The team is winning the game.
c) The team wins the game.
d) The team win the game.

Answer: b) The team is winning the game. Explanation: When "team" is considered a singular entity, the verb should be singular too.

963. Which sentence correctly uses a colon?
a) There are three things you need to make a sandwich: bread, meat, and cheese.
b) There are three things you need to make a sandwich, bread, meat, and cheese.
c) There are three things you need to make a sandwich bread, meat, and cheese.
d) There are three things you need to make a sandwich; bread, meat, and cheese.

Answer: a) There are three things you need to make a sandwich: bread, meat, and cheese. Explanation: A colon is used to introduce a list.

964. Which of the following sentences is grammatically correct?
a) I ain't got no pencils.
b) I don't got no pencils.
c) I haven't any pencils.
d) I doesn't have any pencils.

Answer: c) I haven't any pencils. Explanation: This is the correct use of negative construction in English.

965. Which sentence correctly uses a subordinating conjunction?
a) I like to read and write.
b) I like to read, yet I don't like to write.
c) I like to read, because I learn new words.
d) I like to read but not to write.

Answer: c) I like to read, because I learn new words. Explanation: "Because" is a subordinating conjunction used to show cause and effect.

966. What is the correct contraction for "we are"?
a) we're
b) were
c) we're
d) were'

Answer: a) we're. Explanation: The contraction for "we are" is "we're."

967. Which of the following is a correct plural form of "goose"?
a) Gooses
b) Geese
c) Goos
d) Goosen

Answer: b) Geese. Explanation: The correct plural form of "goose" is "geese."

968. What kind of clause is underlined in this sentence: I went to the park, where I saw a squirrel.
a) Independent clause
b) Dependent clause
c) Noun clause
d) Adverbial clause

Answer: d) Adverbial clause. Explanation: "Where I saw a squirrel" modifies the verb "went" in the independent clause, providing additional information about the location.

969. Which of the following sentences uses a semicolon correctly?
a) The weather is nice today; I am going to the beach.
b) The weather is nice today, I am going to the beach;
c) The weather is nice today; and I am going to the beach.
d) The weather is nice today I am going to the beach;

Answer: a) The weather is nice today; I am going to the beach. Explanation: A semicolon is used to connect two closely related independent clauses.

970. What does the prefix 'un-' mean in the word 'unhappy'?
a) Before
b) Not
c) Very
d) Again

Answer: b) Not. Explanation: The prefix 'un-' typically gives the word it precedes the opposite meaning.

971. Which of the following sentences is in the future perfect tense?
a) I will have finished my homework by dinner.
b) I have finished my homework.
c) I had finished my homework.
d) I will finish my homework.

Answer: a) I will have finished my homework by dinner. Explanation: The future perfect tense uses "will have" plus the past participle of a verb.

972. Which sentence correctly uses their, there, they're?
a) Their going to their house over there.
b) They're going to their house over there.
c) There going to they're house over there.
d) They're going to there house over there.

Answer: b) They're going to their house over there. Explanation: 'They're' is a contraction of 'they are', 'their' shows possession, and 'there' refers to a place.

973. What is the past participle of "drink"?
a) Drunk
b) Drank
c) Drinked
d) Drinking

Answer: a) Drunk. Explanation: The past participle of "drink" is "drunk."

974. Which of the following sentences is in the passive voice?
a) The dog chased the cat.
b) The cat was chased by the dog.
c) The cat chased the dog.
d) The dog was chased by the cat.

Answer: b) The cat was chased by the dog. Explanation: The passive voice occurs when the subject of the sentence is acted upon by the verb.

975. In which sentence is the word "write" used correctly?
a) I need to right a report for work.
b) Right now, I am writing a report for work.
c) I am going to right a report for work.
d) I have to write a report for work.

Answer: d) I have to write a report for work. Explanation: The verb "write" means to inscribe words, sentences, or symbols on a surface.

976. Which of the following sentences correctly uses whom?
a) Whom did you say that was?
b) To whom was the letter written?
c) Who did you give the book to?
d) Who's book is this?

Answer: b) To whom was the letter written? Explanation: "Whom" is used as the object of a verb or preposition.

977. What does the word "retroactive" mean?
a) Pertaining to the past
b) Acting in reverse
c) Applying to a date prior to enactment
d) To activate again

Answer: c) Applying to a date prior to enactment. Explanation: "Retroactive" refers to something extending in scope or effect to a prior time or to conditions that existed or originated in the past.

978. Which word completes this analogy: Cautious is to reckless as brave is to _____.
a) Cowardly
b) Foolish
c) Adventurous
d) Courageous

Answer: a) Cowardly. Explanation: The relationship is one of opposites: Cautious is the opposite of reckless, and brave is the opposite of cowardly.

979. Which of the following words is spelled incorrectly?
a) Occurrence
b) Comittee
c) Privilege
d) Schedule

Answer: b) Comittee. Explanation: The correct spelling is "committee."

980. In which sentence is the word "principal" used correctly?
a) The principal of the school is very strict.
b) The principal reason for my visit is to see the art exhibit.
c) Both a and b
d) None of the above

Answer: c) Both a and b. Explanation: "Principal" can be used as both a noun (referring to the head of a school) and an adjective (meaning the most important).

981. Which of the following words is an antonym for "covert"?
a) Secret
b) Overt
c) Stealthy
d) Concealed

Answer: b) Overt. Explanation: "Overt" is the opposite of "covert," which means not openly acknowledged or displayed.

982. Identify the part of speech of the underlined word in this sentence: The flowers bloomed beautifully in the garden.
a) Adverb
b) Adjective
c) Noun
d) Verb

Answer: a) Adverb. Explanation: "Beautifully" is an adverb because it describes how the flowers bloomed.

983. Which of the following sentences correctly uses a comma?
a) My favorite foods are pizza pasta and sushi.
b) My favorite foods are, pizza, pasta and sushi.
c) My favorite foods are pizza, pasta, and sushi.
d) My favorite, foods are pizza pasta and sushi.

Answer: c) My favorite foods are pizza, pasta, and sushi. Explanation: Commas are used to separate items in a list.

984. What does the prefix "inter-" mean in the word "interstate"?
a) Above
b) Between
c) Under
d) Around

Answer: b) Between. Explanation: The prefix "inter-" typically signifies "between."

985. What kind of sentence is this: Even though it was raining, we decided to go for a walk.
a) Simple sentence
b) Compound sentence
c) Complex sentence
d) Compound-complex sentence

Answer: c) Complex sentence. Explanation: This is a complex sentence because it contains an independent clause ("we decided to go for a walk") and a dependent clause ("even though it was raining").

986. Which of the following sentences demonstrates correct subject-verb agreement?
a) The team of researchers are presenting their findings.
b) The team of researchers is presenting their findings.
c) Neither of the girls are ready for the game.
d) Neither of the girls is ready for the games.

Answer: b) The team of researchers is presenting their findings. Explanation: When a singular noun is preceded by "of," the verb should agree with the singular noun ("team"), not what follows "of."

987. Which of the following is the correct plural form of the word "cactus"?
a) Cacti
b) Cactuses
c) Cactus's
d) Cactus

Answer: a) Cacti. Explanation: The word "cactus" is derived from Latin, and its correct plural form is "cacti," though "cactuses" is also accepted in English.

988. In the sentence "My dog chased its tail," what is the function of the word "its"?
a) Noun
b) Verb
c) Pronoun
d) Adverb

Answer: c) Pronoun. Explanation: "Its" is a possessive pronoun in this sentence, referring back to "my dog."

989. What does the prefix "sub-" mean in the word "submarine"?
a) Above
b) Below
c) In between
d) Under

Answer: d) Under. Explanation: The prefix "sub-" generally means "under" or "below."

990. Which of the following sentences correctly uses quotation marks?
a) My favorite book is "To Kill a Mockingbird."
b) My favorite book is To Kill a Mockingbird.
c) My favorite book is "To Kill a Mockingbird".
d) My favorite book is, "To Kill a Mockingbird."

Answer: a) My favorite book is "To Kill a Mockingbird." Explanation: Quotation marks are used to indicate titles of books, articles, songs, and other works of art.

991. In which sentence is the word "effect" used correctly?
a) The drug had an immediate effect on the patient.
b) The drug had an immediate affect on the patient.
c) The effect of the sun was immediate.
d) Both a and c

Answer: d) Both a and c. Explanation: "Effect" as a noun typically means a result or an outcome.

992. Which of the following sentences is written in the active voice?
a) The game was won by the team.
b) The team won the game.
c) The game is being played by the team.
d) The game was being played by the team.

Answer: b) The team won the game. Explanation: Active voice occurs when the subject of the sentence performs the action, as in "The team won the game."

993. In the sentence "I want to go to the store, but I have no car," what is the conjunction?
a) Want
b) To
c) But
d) Have

Answer: c) But. Explanation: "But" is a conjunction used to connect two clauses in the sentence.

994. In the sentence "She is a very talented dancer," what is the adjective?
a) She
b) Is
c) Very
d) Talented

Answer: d) Talented. Explanation: "Talented" is an adjective because it describes a noun (dancer).

995. What is the past tense of the verb "to swim"?
a) Swimmed
b) Swam
c) Swum
d) Swims

Answer: b) Swam. Explanation: The past tense of "to swim" is "swam."

996. Which of the following sentences contains a dangling modifier?
a) Walking down the street, the trees were beautiful.
b) I saw a beautiful bird while walking down the street.
c) The trees were beautiful, covered in blossoms.
d) Covered in blossoms, the trees were beautiful.

Answer: a) Walking down the street, the trees were beautiful. Explanation: In this sentence, "Walking down the street" is a dangling modifier because it does not correctly modify any word in the sentence.

997. Which of the following words is a homonym for "flower"?
a) Flour
b) Flaw
c) Flier
d) Flow

Answer: a) Flour. Explanation: Homonyms are words that are pronounced the same but have different meanings. "Flower" and "flour" are homonyms.

998. In the sentence "John is taller than me," which pronoun should replace "me" to make the sentence grammatically correct?
a) I
b) He
c) Him
d) It

Answer: a) I. Explanation: The correct comparative form is "John is taller than I (am)," where "am" is often omitted in informal language.

999. The sentence "I wish I was a bird" should be corrected to:
a) I wish I were a bird
b) I wish I will be a bird
c) I wish I would be a bird
d) The sentence is correct as is

Answer: a) I wish I were a bird. Explanation: In English, we use "were" instead of "was" after "wish" and phrases that suggest something that is unlikely or not true.

1000. What is the correct plural form of the word "mouse"?
a) Mice
b) Mouses
c) Mouse's
d) Mouce

Answer: a) Mice. Explanation: The plural of "mouse" is "mice."

1001. In which of the following sentences is "there" used as a pronoun?
a) There are many people at the party.
b) The cat is over there.
c) There is no need to be upset.
d) Both a and c

Answer: d) Both a and c. Explanation: "There" can be used as a pronoun to introduce a sentence or clause, as seen in the examples.

1002. Which of the following sentences uses a semi-colon correctly?
a) I have a big test tomorrow; I can't go to the party.
b) I have a big test tomorrow, I can't go to the party.
c) I have a big test tomorrow; and I can't go to the party.
d) I have a big test tomorrow; because I can't go to the party.

Answer: a) I have a big test tomorrow; I can't go to the party. Explanation: A semi-colon is used to connect two independent clauses.

1003. Which sentence is an example of hyperbole?
a) She runs faster than the wind.
b) He is as tall as a tree.
c) I have told you a million times.
d) Your bag weighs a ton.

Answer: c) I have told you a million times. Explanation: Hyperbole is an exaggerated statement not meant to be taken literally.

1004. What is the past participle of the verb "to go"?
a) Gone
b) Goes
c) Went
d) Going

Answer: a) Gone. Explanation: The past participle of "to go" is "gone."

1005. In the sentence "The house, which is old, is in the countryside," what is the function of the phrase "which is old"?
a) Adjective
b) Adverb
c) Interjection
d) Noun

Answer: a) Adjective. Explanation: The phrase "which is old" acts as an adjective, modifying the noun "house."

1006. Which of the following sentences is written in the passive voice?
a) The cat chased the mouse.
b) The mouse was chased by the cat.
c) She painted a beautiful picture.
d) They ate all the food.

Answer: b) The mouse was chased by the cat. Explanation: In passive voice, the object of the action becomes the subject of the sentence.

1007. Which of the following sentences is a fragment?
a) She went to the store.
b) Bought a loaf of bread.
c) He read a book in the park.
d) The cat is sleeping on the mat.

Answer: b) Bought a loaf of bread. Explanation: This sentence is a fragment because it lacks a subject.

1008. Which of the following sentences contains an example of a metaphor?
a) His smile is as bright as the sun.
b) She swims like a fish.
c) Life is a rollercoaster.
d) The snow is a white blanket.

Answer: c) Life is a rollercoaster. Explanation: A metaphor is a figure of speech that makes a comparison by directly relating one thing to another unrelated thing. In this case, life is compared to a rollercoaster.

1009. What is the correct way to combine these two sentences: "I love reading. I love writing"?
a) I love reading and I love writing.
b) I love reading, I love writing.
c) I love reading; I love writing.
d) Both a and c

Answer: d) Both a and c. Explanation: Both options create grammatically correct sentences. Option b creates a run-on sentence, which is incorrect.

1010. Which of the following words is a synonym for "happy"?
a) Elated
b) Sad
c) Angry
d) Depressed

Answer: a) Elated. Explanation: Elated is a synonym for happy, which means filled with happiness and enthusiasm.

1011. In the sentence "The dog's tail wagged rapidly," which word is the adverb?
a) Dog's
b) Tail
c) Wagged
d) Rapidly

Answer: d) Rapidly. Explanation: An adverb is a word that describes a verb, an adjective, or other adverbs. "Rapidly" is describing how the tail wagged, so it is the adverb in this sentence.

1012. Choose the correct verb tense for the sentence: "By the time we get there, the store _____."
a) Will close
b) Will have closed
c) Has closed
d) Close

Answer: b) Will have closed. Explanation: "Will have closed" is the correct future perfect tense verb form to use in this sentence.

1013. What is the past tense of the verb "to drive"?
a) Drove
b) Driven
c) Drives
d) Driving

Answer: a) Drove. Explanation: The past tense of "to drive" is "drove."

1014. Which of the following words is the antonym of "beautiful"?
a) Attractive
b) Lovely
c) Ugly
d) Pretty

Answer: c) Ugly. Explanation: An antonym is a word that has the opposite meaning of another word. "Ugly" is the opposite of "beautiful."

1015. What type of sentence is this: "If it's sunny, we'll go to the park."?
a) Declarative
b) Interrogative
c) Exclamatory
d) Conditional

Answer: d) Conditional. Explanation: This is a conditional sentence because it sets up a condition (if it's sunny) and the result of that condition (we'll go to the park).

1016. In the sentence "The teacher gave the students the books," what is the indirect object?
a) Teacher
b) Gave
c) Students
d) Books

Answer: c) Students. Explanation: The indirect object is the person or thing who receives the direct object. In this case, "the students" are receiving "the books."

1017. Which of the following is not a common factor of 20 and 30?
a) 2
b) 5
c) 10
d) 7

Answer: d) 7. Explanation: A common factor is a number that divides exactly into two or more other numbers. The common factors of 20 and 30 are 1, 2, 5, and 10.

1018. Which is the first step in the scientific method?
a) Hypothesis
b) Observation
c) Experiment
d) Conclusion

Answer: b) Observation. Explanation: The first step of the scientific method is observation. This is when you notice and describe what is happening, which forms the basis for the next steps.

1019. Which of the following words is a synonym for "sad"?
a) Joyful
b) Glee
c) Happy
d) Mournful

Answer: d) Mournful. Explanation: A synonym is a word or phrase that means exactly or nearly the same as another word or phrase. 'Mournful' has a similar meaning to 'sad.'

1020. Which body system is responsible for transporting nutrients, hormones, and gases to cells?
a) Digestive system
b) Circulatory system
c) Respiratory system
d) Nervous system

Answer: b) Circulatory system. Explanation: The circulatory system is responsible for transporting nutrients, hormones, and gases to cells.

1021. In the following sentence, what is the antecedent of the pronoun "it"? "I can't believe it's already the end of the year; it went by so fast!"
a) Year
b) Believe
c) End
d) Fast

Answer: a) Year. Explanation: An antecedent is a word, phrase, clause, or sentence to which another word (especially a following relative pronoun) refers. In this case, 'it' is referring to 'year.'

1022. Which of the following is an example of a rational number?
a) √2
b) π
c) 2/3
d) √-1

Answer: c) 2/3. Explanation: Rational numbers can be expressed as a fraction where both the numerator and the denominator are integers.

1023. Which of the following is an example of personification?
a) The wind whispered through the trees.
b) She runs like a gazelle.
c) He is as brave as a lion.
d) Her eyes are stars.

Answer: a) The wind whispered through the trees. Explanation: Personification is a figure of speech where non-human objects are described as having human qualities.

1024. Which of the following sentences uses a preposition incorrectly?
a) The book is on the table.
b) I will meet you at six o'clock.
c) She arrived to the party late.
d) We are going for a walk.

Answer: c) She arrived to the party late. Explanation: The correct preposition to use with "arrived" in this context is "at."

1025. Which form of cellular respiration generates the most ATP?
a) Glycolysis
b) Krebs Cycle
c) Electron Transport Chain
d) Fermentation

Answer: c) Electron Transport Chain. Explanation: The electron transport chain is the final stage of aerobic respiration and it generates the most ATP.

1026. Which of the following best describes the main idea of a paragraph?
a) The first sentence of the paragraph
b) The most important point the author wants to make
c) A sentence that describes the conclusion
d) The supporting details that provide evidence

Answer: b) The most important point the author wants to make.

1027. Which organ is responsible for detoxifying chemicals and metabolizing drugs in the body?
a) The kidneys
b) The heart
c) The liver
d) The lungs

Answer: c) The liver. Explanation: The liver has the primary role of detoxifying chemicals and metabolizing drugs in the body, keeping the body free from harmful substances.

1028. In the following sentence, which is the dependent clause? "Although it was raining, we decided to go out for a walk."
a) Although it was raining
b) we decided to go out for a walk
c) it was raining
d) for a walk

Answer: a) Although it was raining. Explanation: A dependent clause is a group of words with a subject and a verb. It does not express a complete thought so it is not a sentence and can't stand alone.

1029. Solve for x: 5x - 7 = 18
a) x = 3
b) x = 5
c) x = 4
d) x = 7

Answer: c) x = 4. Explanation: By adding 7 to both sides of the equation, we get 5x = 25. Dividing both sides by 5 gives x = 4.

1030. What is the primary function of white blood cells?
a) Carrying oxygen
b) Clotting blood
c) Fighting infection
d) Regulating body temperature

Answer: c) Fighting infection. Explanation: The primary function of white blood cells is to fight off infection and disease in the body.

1031. Which of the following sentences uses correct punctuation?
a) We're going to the beach are you coming with us.
b) We're going to the beach; are you coming with us?
c) We're going to the beach, are you, coming with us.
d) We're going to the beach, are you coming with us.

Answer: b) We're going to the beach; are you coming with us? Explanation: The semicolon correctly separates the two independent clauses, and the question mark appropriately punctuates the question.

1032. Which of the following numbers is not a prime number?
a) 7
b) 13
c) 15
d) 17

Answer: c) 15. Explanation: A prime number is a natural number greater than 1 that has no positive divisors other than 1 and itself. 15 is not a prime number because it has divisors other than 1 and itself (3 and 5).

1033. Which of the following terms is a figure of speech that compares two things by using "like" or "as"?
a) Metaphor
b) Hyperbole
c) Simile
d) Alliteration

Answer: c) Simile. Explanation: A simile is a figure of speech that makes a comparison, showing similarities between two different things using "like" or "as".

1034. What phase of mitosis is characterized by the alignment of chromosomes along the middle of the cell?
a) Prophase
b) Metaphase
c) Anaphase
d) Telophase

Answer: b) Metaphase. Explanation: During metaphase, the chromosomes align in the middle of the cell, preparing for separation into the two daughter cells.

1035. Which of the following passages is an example of first-person narration?
a) "She walked down the aisle, her heart pounding in her chest."
b) "You need to finish your homework before going to the party."
c) "I watched the sun set over the mountains, feeling a sense of peace."
d) "Walking down the street, they spotted a familiar face."

Answer: c) "I watched the sun set over the mountains, feeling a sense of peace." Explanation: The use of "I" indicates first-person narration.

1036. In the equation of a line y = mx + b, what does the "m" represent?
a) The y-intercept
b) The x-intercept
c) The slope
d) The distance from the origin

Answer: c) The slope. Explanation: In the equation of a line, y = mx + b, "m" represents the slope of the line.

1037. The density of a substance is calculated by:
a) Mass times Volume
b) Mass divided by Volume
c) Volume divided by Mass
d) Volume times Mass

Answer: b) Mass divided by Volume. Explanation: Density is calculated by dividing the mass of a substance by its volume.

1038. Which of the following words correctly completes the sentence: "The patient's symptoms were _____."
a) effecting his daily activities
b) affecting his daily activities
c) infecting his daily activities
d) effacing his daily activities

Answer: b) affecting his daily activities. Explanation: 'Affecting' is the correct verb to use when referring to something influencing someone or something else.

1039. If a solution has a pH of 9, it is:
a) Neutral
b) Acidic
c) Basic
d) Not enough information to tell

Answer: c) Basic. Explanation: A solution with a pH above 7 is considered basic or alkaline.

1040. In the following sentence, which is the main subject? "The quick brown fox jumps over the lazy dog."
a) The quick brown fox
b) jumps
c) over
d) the lazy dog

Answer: a) The quick brown fox. Explanation: The main subject of a sentence is the person, place, thing, or idea that is doing or being something. Here, "The quick brown fox" is the subject.

1041. Solve for x: 4x + 2 = 18
a) x = 4
b) x = 3
c) x = 5
d) x = 8

Answer: b) x = 3. Explanation: By subtracting 2 from both sides and then dividing by 4, we find that x = 3.

1042. Which term best describes the relationship between two organisms where one benefits and the other is not significantly harmed or helped?
a) Parasitism
b) Mutualism
c) Commensalism
d) Symbiosis

Answer: c) Commensalism. Explanation: Commensalism describes a relationship where one organism benefits but the other is neither harmed nor helped.

1043. Which of the following sentences uses an adverb correctly?
a) He runs quick.
b) She sings beautifully.
c) He looks sadly.
d) They dance good.

Answer: b) She sings beautifully. Explanation: An adverb modifies a verb, an adjective, or another adverb. In this sentence, 'beautifully' is an adverb that modifies the verb 'sings'.

1044. If a = 3 and b = 4, what is the value of 2a + b?
a) 8
b) 10
c) 14
d) 6

Answer: b) 10. Explanation: Substituting the given values, we have 2*3 + 4 = 6 + 4 = 10.

1045. Which type of cell division results in daughter cells with half the number of chromosomes of the parent cell?
a) Mitosis
b) Meiosis
c) Cytokinesis
d) Binary fission

Answer: b) Meiosis. Explanation: Meiosis is a type of cell division that reduces the number of chromosomes in the parent cell by half and produces four gamete cells.

1046. In a sentence, the verb typically expresses:
a) A state of being
b) An action
c) Either a state of being or an action
d) The object of the sentence

Answer: c) Either a state of being or an action. Explanation: Verbs can express both states of being (like 'is', 'are', 'was', 'were') and actions (like 'run', 'jump', 'think').

1047. The process by which water vapor changes from a gas to a liquid is known as:
a) Evaporation
b) Condensation
c) Sublimation
d) Transpiration

Answer: b) Condensation. Explanation: Condensation is the process by which water vapor in the air is changed into liquid water.

1048. In mathematics, a variable often used to represent an unknown value is:
a) A number
b) A letter
c) A symbol
d) A word

Answer: b) A letter. Explanation: In mathematics, letters are often used to represent variables, which can stand for unknown values.

1049. Select the correctly spelled word:
a) Embarrassment
b) Embarrasment
c) Embarrassmant
d) Embarrasement

Answer: a) Embarrassment. Explanation: The correct spelling is 'Embarrassment'.

1050. What is the primary role of the Golgi apparatus in cells?
a) Protein synthesis
b) DNA replication
c) Modifying, sorting and packaging of proteins
d) Breakdown of waste materials

Answer: c) Modifying, sorting and packaging of proteins. Explanation: The Golgi apparatus modifies, sorts, and packages proteins for secretion or use within the cell.

1051. Identify the noun in the following sentence: "The boy threw the ball."
a) The
b) Boy
c) Threw
d) Ball

Answer: d) Ball. Explanation: A noun is a word that represents a person, place, thing, or idea. In this sentence, 'ball' is a thing and therefore is a noun.

1052. In mathematics, what does the term 'integer' refer to?
a) A number that can be written without a fractional component
b) A number that is not a whole number
c) A number with a fractional component
d) A negative number

Answer: a) A number that can be written without a fractional component. Explanation: Integers include all whole numbers, both positive and negative, and zero.

1053. Which of the following is an example of a simile?
a) The wind whispered through the trees.
b) He was as brave as a lion.
c) Time is a thief.
d) She's a shining star.

Answer: b) He was as brave as a lion. Explanation: A simile is a figure of speech that compares two unlike things using the words 'like' or 'as'.

1054. Which layer of the Earth is located immediately below the crust?
a) Core
b) Mantle
c) Outer core
d) Inner core

Answer: b) Mantle. Explanation: The Earth's mantle is located directly beneath the crust.

1055. Which of the following is an example of a complex sentence?
a) I like tea.
b) I like tea because it wakes me up in the morning.
c) I like tea and coffee.
d) Although I like tea, I prefer coffee in the morning.

Answer: d) Although I like tea, I prefer coffee in the morning. Explanation: A complex sentence contains one independent clause and at least one dependent clause.

1056. Solve for y: 2y - 6 = 8
a) y = 7
b) y = 5
c) y = 3
d) y = 2

Answer: b) y = 5. Explanation: By adding 6 to both sides and then dividing by 2, we find that y = 5.

1057. Identify the adjective in the following sentence: "The red ball bounced across the green lawn."
a) Ball
b) Bounced
c) Red
d) Lawn

Answer: c) Red. Explanation: An adjective is a word that describes a noun. In this sentence, 'red' is describing the noun 'ball,' therefore it is the adjective.

1058. Which term refers to the amount of space an object occupies?
a) Mass
b) Volume
c) Density
d) Weight

Answer: b) Volume. Explanation: Volume refers to the quantity of three-dimensional space occupied by a substance or enclosed by a surface.

1059. When a caterpillar changes into a butterfly, it undergoes:
a) Metamorphosis
b) Mutation
c) Fission
d) Evolution

Answer: a) Metamorphosis. Explanation: Metamorphosis is a process by which an animal physically develops after birth or hatching, often involving a conspicuous and relatively abrupt change.

1060. Choose the option that best fits the blank: "Despite his _____, he couldn't resist the temptation of the cookie jar."
a) satiety
b) hunger
c) thirst
d) fatigue

Answer: a) satiety. Explanation: 'Satiety' refers to the state of being full or gratified to or beyond the point of satisfaction.

1061. Solve the equation: $5x + 2 = 12$
a) $x = 1$
b) $x = 2$
c) $x = 3$
d) $x = 4$

Answer: b) $x = 2$. Explanation: If you subtract 2 from both sides, you get $5x = 10$. Dividing both sides by 5 gives $x = 2$.

1062. In the human body, which organ is primarily responsible for detoxification?
a) Heart
b) Kidney
c) Liver
d) Lung

Answer: c) Liver. Explanation: The liver's main job is to filter the blood coming from the digestive tract, before passing it to the rest of the body.

1063. Which of the following is an example of a metaphor?
a) Her laughter was music to his ears.
b) He swims like a fish.
c) She is as brave as a lion.
d) Time flies when you're having fun.

Answer: a) Her laughter was music to his ears. Explanation: A metaphor is a figure of speech that refers to one thing by mentioning another thing. Here, her laughter is not literally music, but is being compared to music because it is pleasant to hear.

1064. Which term refers to the number of protons in the nucleus of an atom?
a) Atomic number
b) Atomic mass
c) Isotope
d) Neutron number

Answer: a) Atomic number. Explanation: The atomic number of a chemical element is the number of protons found in the nucleus of an atom.

1065. Which type of text is intended to persuade the reader to adopt a particular viewpoint?
a) Descriptive
b) Narrative
c) Expository
d) Argumentative

Answer: d) Argumentative. Explanation: Argumentative texts are intended to convince the reader of a particular point of view.

1066. The sum of all angles in a triangle is equal to:
a) 90 degrees
b) 180 degrees
c) 270 degrees
d) 360 degrees

Answer: b) 180 degrees. Explanation: In a triangle, the sum of all the internal angles is always equal to 180 degrees.

1067. "The knee is _____ to the ankle."
a) distal
b) lateral
c) superior
d) proximal

Answer: a) distal
Explanation: The term 'distal' in anatomy is used to describe something that is further away from the center of the body, or the point of attachment. In this case, the knee is further away from the center of the body when compared to the ankle. Hence, the knee is distal to the ankle.

1068. When working with algebraic equations, what does the distributive property state?
a) $a(b + c) = ab + ac$
b) $a(b - c) = ab - ac$
c) $a + (b + c) = (a + b) + c$
d) $a(b/c) = (ab)/c$

Answer: a) a(b + c) = ab + ac
Explanation: The distributive property states that the multiplication of a number and the sum of two others is equal to the sum of the multiplication of the number and each of the two others separately.

1069. In a patient with Type 2 diabetes, which of the following would you expect to find in a routine blood test?
a) Elevated levels of insulin
b) Reduced levels of glucose
c) Elevated levels of glucose
d) Reduced levels of insulin

Answer: c) Elevated levels of glucose
Explanation: Type 2 diabetes is characterized by high levels of sugar (glucose) in the blood. This is due to the body's resistance to the effects of insulin and/or insufficient insulin production.

1070. What does an adverb typically modify?
a) A noun
b) A verb
c) An adjective
d) A and C

Answer: b) A verb
Explanation: An adverb is a word that modifies a verb, an adjective, or another adverb. But most commonly, it modifies a verb.

1071. The human body is composed of how many types of tissue?
a) 2
b) 4
c) 5
d) 3

Answer: b) 4
Explanation: The human body is made up of four basic types of tissue: epithelial, connective, muscle, and nervous tissue.

1072. Which of the following is a correctly punctuated compound sentence?
a) I am studying for the TEAS exam it is quite challenging.
b) I am studying for the TEAS exam, it is quite challenging.
c) I am studying for the TEAS exam; it is quite challenging.
d) I am studying for the TEAS exam: it is quite challenging.

Answer: c) I am studying for the TEAS exam; it is quite challenging.
Explanation: A compound sentence is made up of two or more independent clauses that are joined using a conjunction, semicolon, or comma. In this case, the semicolon correctly connects the two independent clauses.

1073. Which of the following is an example of a hyperbola?
a) $y = x^2$
b) $y = 1/x$
c) $y = x^3$
d) $y = x$

Answer: b) $y = 1/x$
Explanation: A hyperbola is a type of smooth curve lying in a plane, defined by its geometric properties. In the equation $y = 1/x$, as x approaches 0 from the right (positive side), y increases without bound (tends to infinity). As x approaches 0 from the left (negative side), y decreases without bound (tends to negative infinity).

1074. In the circulatory system, what does the right ventricle do?
a) It pumps oxygenated blood to the body.
b) It pumps deoxygenated blood to the lungs.
c) It receives oxygenated blood from the lungs.
d) It receives deoxygenated blood from the body.

Answer: b) It pumps deoxygenated blood to the lungs.
Explanation: The right ventricle is one of the four chambers of the heart. It receives deoxygenated blood from the right atrium and pumps it under low pressure into the lungs for oxygenation.

1075. Complete the sentence with the correct form of the verb: "If I _____ more time, I would study all the subjects."
a) had
b) have
c) has
d) having

Answer: a) had
Explanation: In English, we use "If I had" for hypothetical or unreal conditions in the present or future.

1076. Which of the following explains the principle of conservation of energy?
a) Energy cannot be created or destroyed, but only changed from one form into another.
b) The total amount of energy in an isolated system remains constant over time.
c) Both A and B.
d) None of the above.

Answer: c) Both A and B.
Explanation: The principle of conservation of energy states that the total energy of an isolated system remains constant—it is said to be conserved over time. This law means that energy can neither be created nor destroyed; rather, it can only be transformed or transferred from one form to another.

1077. "Identifying the main idea of a passage can greatly assist in _____."
a) finding supporting details
b) understanding the author's intent
c) summarizing the content
d) all of the above

Answer: d) all of the above.
Explanation: Identifying the main idea of a passage assists in finding supporting details, understanding the author's intent, and summarizing the content. It helps provide a clear picture of the message the author is trying to convey.

1078. Which of the following is the solution to the equation $3x - 5 = 16$?
a) $x = 3$
b) $x = 5$
c) $x = 7$
d) $x = 8$

Answer: c) $x = 7$
Explanation: To solve for x, first add 5 to both sides of the equation to get $3x = 21$. Then divide both sides by 3 to get $x = 7$.

1079. What is the role of the ribosomes in a cell?
a) It stores DNA
b) It assists in cell division
c) It produces proteins
d) It controls cell movement

Answer: c) It produces proteins
Explanation: The primary function of ribosomes in a cell is to produce proteins, which is vital for the cell's operations.

1080. Identify the adverb in the following sentence: "She quickly ran to the store."
a) she
b) quickly
c) ran
d) store

Answer: b) quickly
Explanation: In the given sentence, 'quickly' is the adverb. Adverbs modify verbs, adjectives, or other adverbs, and in this case, 'quickly' is modifying the verb 'ran'.

1081. Which of the following body systems is responsible for the removal of waste?
a) Nervous system
b) Circulatory system
c) Respiratory system
d) Excretory system

Answer: d) Excretory system
Explanation: The excretory system is primarily responsible for the removal of waste products from the body.

1082. "In a non-fiction piece of writing, a writer's main argument is usually found in the _____."
a) conclusion
b) introduction
c) body paragraphs
d) thesis statement

Answer: d) thesis statement
Explanation: The thesis statement, usually found in the introduction of a non-fiction piece of writing, presents the writer's main argument. It gives the reader a clear understanding of what the piece will be discussing.

1083. The solution to the equation $4x + 3 = 27$ is:
a) $x = 4$
b) $x = 5$
c) $x = 6$
d) $x = 7$

Answer: c) $x = 6$
Explanation: To solve for x, first subtract 3 from both sides of the equation to get $4x = 24$. Then divide both sides by 4 to get $x = 6$.

1084. The human body's first line of defense against disease-causing organisms is the:
a) immune system
b) respiratory system
c) skin
d) nervous system

Answer: c) skin
Explanation: The skin acts as a physical barrier, preventing pathogens from entering the body, making it the body's first line of defense against disease-caising organisms.

1085. Which word in the following sentence is an adverb: "The cat quietly crept up on the unsuspecting bird."
a) cat
b) quietly
c) crept
d) bird

Answer: b) quietly
Explanation: In the given sentence, 'quietly' is the adverb as it is modifying the verb 'crept' by explaining how the action was performed.

1086. Which body system regulates and controls growth, development, and metabolism?
a) The nervous system
b) The endocrine system
c) The excretory system
d) The circulatory system

Answer: b) The endocrine system
Explanation: The endocrine system, through the secretion of hormones, regulates and controls various functions in the body including growth, development, and metabolism.

1087. Which of the following phrases should be used to correct the following sentence: "I enjoy to play soccer on the weekends."
a) "I enjoyed playing soccer on the weekends."
b) "I enjoy playing soccer on the weekends."
c) "I enjoying to play soccer on the weekends."
d) "I play soccer on the weekends."

Answer: b) "I enjoy playing soccer on the weekends."
Explanation: The verb 'enjoy' is followed by a gerund (-ing form of the verb), not an infinitive (to + verb), so the correct phrase would be "I enjoy playing soccer on the weekends."

1088. Which of the following is not a primary color of light?
a) Red
b) Green
c) Blue
d) Yellow

Answer: d) Yellow
Explanation: The primary colors of light are red, green, and blue. Yellow is not a primary color of light but is instead a secondary color that can be created by mixing red and green light.

1089. The most appropriate transition to add at the beginning of a contrasting paragraph is:
a) "Additionally,"
b) "For instance,"
c) "However,"
d) "In summary,"

Answer: c) "However,"
Explanation: The transitional word "However," signals a contrast or change in direction from the previous point or idea, which is appropriate when beginning a paragraph that presents contrasting information.

1090. The best interpretation of a text's meaning often comes from _____.
a) understanding the historical context in which it was written
b) applying one's personal beliefs to the text
c) relying on a single, literal interpretation
d) reading as quickly as possible

Answer: a) understanding the historical context in which it was written
Explanation: While all interpretations are subject to the reader's perspective, understanding the historical and cultural context in which a text was written often provides deeper insights into its intended meaning.

1091. What type of bond occurs when electrons are shared between atoms?
a) Ionic bond
b) Covalent bond
c) Hydrogen bond
d) Metallic bond

Answer: b) Covalent bond
Explanation: Covalent bonds occur when electrons are shared between atoms. This sharing allows each atom to reach a stable electron configuration.

1092. "In a properly structured paragraph, the topic sentence usually appears _____."
a) at the end
b) in the middle
c) at the beginning
d) any position

Answer: c) at the beginning
Explanation: The topic sentence is typically the first sentence of a paragraph and it introduces the main idea to be discussed in the paragraph.

1093. Find the value of x if 5x - 12 = 8.
a) x = 4
b) x = 5
c) x = 3
d) x = 6

Answer: a) x = 4
Explanation: To find the value of x, you first add 12 to both sides of the equation to get 5x = 20. Then, you divide both sides by 5 to get x = 4.

1094. The smallest unit of life that can function independently is a(n):
a) organ
b) cell
c) tissue
d) organism

Answer: b) cell
Explanation: The cell is the smallest unit of life that can function independently. It is the basic structural, functional, and biological unit of all known organisms.

1095. Which of the following best identifies the verb in the sentence: "The dog barked loudly at the mailman."
a) dog
b) barked
c) loudly
d) mailman

Answer: b) barked
Explanation: In this sentence, 'barked' is the verb as it describes the action being performed by the subject, the dog.

1096. Which body system breaks down food into nutrients that can be used by the body?
a) The nervous system
b) The circulatory system
c) The digestive system
d) The endocrine system

Answer: c) The digestive system
Explanation: The digestive system is responsible for breaking down food into nutrients that the body can use for energy, growth, and cell repair.

1097. The phrase "an unkind word" should replace which words in the following sentence: "She spoke a word that wasn't nice."
a) She spoke
b) a word
c) that wasn't nice
d) spoke a word

Answer: c) that wasn't nice
Explanation: The phrase "that wasn't nice" can be replaced with "an unkind word" to make the sentence: "She spoke an unkind word."

1098. The atomic number of an element represents the number of:
a) Protons in the nucleus
b) Neutrons in the nucleus
c) Electrons in the outermost shell
d) Total number of particles in the nucleus

Answer: a) Protons in the nucleus
Explanation: The atomic number of an element corresponds to the number of protons in its nucleus.

1099. The best way to make the conclusion of an essay impactful is to _____.
a) introduce a new idea
b) summarize the main points
c) question the reader
d) contradict the thesis statement

Answer: b) summarize the main points
Explanation: In the conclusion of an essay, summarizing the main points can help reaffirm the argument for the reader, making it more impactful.

1100. The best way to find the main idea of a reading passage is to _____.
a) read the first sentence of every paragraph
b) read the conclusion of the passage
c) skim through the entire passage quickly
d) understand the context of the passage

Answer: d) understand the context of the passage
Explanation: Understanding the context of a passage often provides the best insight into the main idea. This typically involves a more careful and detailed reading of the entire passage.

1101. A pH value of 7 represents a _____ solution.
a) highly acidic
b) slightly acidic
c) neutral
d) highly basic

Answer: c) neutral
Explanation: A pH value of 7 indicates a neutral solution, neither acidic nor basic.

1102. "What is the common term for the bones that comprise the axial skeleton?"
a) Vertebrae
b) Cranium
c) Skull and spine
d) Pelvis and femur

Answer: c) Skull and spine
Explanation: The axial skeleton is comprised primarily of the skull and spine, along with the rib cage.

1103. Which sentence best uses a semicolon?
a) I have a big test tomorrow; I can't go to the party.
b) I have a big test tomorrow, I can't go to the party.
c) I have a big test tomorrow - I can't go to the party.
d) I have a big test tomorrow and, I can't go to the party.

Answer: a) I have a big test tomorrow; I can't go to the party.
Explanation: Semicolons are used to connect two independent clauses that are closely related in thought.

1104. What is the solution to the equation 2x - 5 = 15?
a) x = 5
b) x = 10
c) x = 7
d) x = 4

Answer: a) x = 5
Explanation: To solve for x, you add 5 to both sides of the equation to get 2x = 20. Then you divide by 2 to get x = 10.

1105. Which organ is responsible for detoxifying chemicals and metabolizing drugs?
a) Kidneys
b) Liver
c) Pancreas
d) Spleen

Answer: b) Liver
Explanation: The liver has many functions, including detoxifying chemicals and metabolizing drugs.

1106. Which literary device is used in this sentence: "The leaves danced in the wind."
a) Metaphor
b) Simile
c) Personification
d) Hyperbole

Answer: c) Personification
Explanation: Personification is a figure of speech in which a thing, an idea or an animal is given human attributes.

1107. Which term refers to the number of square units that covers a shape or figure?
a) Perimeter
b) Area
c) Volume
d) Circumference

Answer: b) Area
Explanation: Area refers to the number of square units that covers a shape or figure.

1108. What type of bond forms when electrons are shared between atoms?
a) Covalent bond
b) Ionic bond
c) Hydrogen bond
d) Metallic bond

Answer: a) Covalent bond
Explanation: A covalent bond is a chemical bond that involves the sharing of electron pairs between atoms.

1109. Which sentence correctly uses the word "their"?
a) Their is a cat in the yard.
b) I can't find their.
c) Their are four apples on the table.
d) Their house is on the corner.

Answer: d) Their house is on the corner.
Explanation: "Their" is a possessive pronoun used to indicate ownership.

1110. What is the main function of white blood cells?
a) Carrying oxygen
b) Blood clotting
c) Fighting infections
d) Transporting nutrients

Answer: c) Fighting infections
Explanation: The primary function of white blood cells, or leukocytes, is to fight infections and disease.

1111. In the given excerpt, the author is primarily concerned with _____.
a) presenting a problem and its solution
b) comparing and contrasting two ideas
c) persuading the reader of a certain viewpoint
d) describing a scene in detail

Answer: This question is not complete without an accompanying excerpt for reference.

1112. Which of the following organs is part of the digestive system?
a) Lungs
b) Kidneys
c) Stomach
d) Brain

Answer: c) Stomach
Explanation: The stomach is part of the digestive system and helps break down food for the body to use.

1113. Identify the verb in the following sentence: "The cat chased the mouse."
a) The
b) Cat
c) Chased
d) Mouse

Answer: c) Chased
Explanation: In this sentence, "chased" is the verb, or the action that the subject (the cat) is performing.

1114. If $x = 3$ and $y = 5$, what is the value of $2x + 3y$?
a) 21
b) 23
c) 25
d) 27

Answer: a) 21
Explanation: Substitute the given values into the expression: 2(3) + 3(5) = 6 + 15 = 21.

1115. Which of the following is an example of a chemical change?
a) Ice melting
b) Sugar dissolving in water
c) A log burning
d) Cutting a piece of paper

Answer: c) A log burning
Explanation: A log burning involves a chemical reaction, making it a chemical change.

1116. Which word is spelled incorrectly in the following sentence? "She recieved a beautiful bouqet of roses."
a) She
b) recieved
c) beautiful
d) bouqet

Answer: b) recieved and d) bouqet
Explanation: The correct spelling is "received" and "bouquet".

1117. What is the range of the data set {3, 7, 10, 12, 15}?
a) 15
b) 12
c) 10
d) 3

Answer: a) 15 - 3 = 12
Explanation: The range of a data set is the difference between the largest and smallest values.

1118. What is the atomic number of an atom with 7 protons, 7 neutrons, and 7 electrons?
a) 7
b) 14
c) 21
d) 28

Answer: a) 7
Explanation: The atomic number of an atom is equal to the number of protons in its nucleus, which in this case is 7.

1119. Which punctuation mark should be used to combine the following two independent clauses? "She wanted to go for a run; She had to finish her homework first."
a) Comma
b) Semicolon
c) Colon
d) Hyphen

Answer: b) Semicolon
Explanation: A semicolon can be used to combine two closely related independent clauses.

1120. The function of the pancreas in the human body includes which of the following?
a) Producing insulin
b) Filtering waste from the blood
c) Producing bile for digestion
d) Pumping blood throughout the body

Answer: a) Producing insulin
Explanation: The pancreas produces insulin, a hormone that regulates the amount of glucose in the body's blood.

1121. Which type of context clue relies on a comparison to describe an unfamiliar word?
a) Definition context clues
b) Synonym context clues
c) Antonym context clues
d) Analogy context clues

Answer: d) Analogy context clues
Explanation: Analogy context clues rely on comparisons or relationships with other words to help infer the meaning of an unfamiliar word.

1122. What is the main function of the circulatory system?
a) Digestion of food
b) Control of body movement
c) Transport of oxygen and nutrients
d) Regulation of body temperature

Answer: c) Transport of oxygen and nutrients
Explanation: The primary function of the circulatory system is to transport oxygen, nutrients, and other substances throughout the body, and to remove waste products.

1123. Which word in the following sentence is an adverb: "She quickly ran to the store."
a) She
b) Quickly
c) Ran
d) Store

Answer: b) Quickly
Explanation: In this sentence, "quickly" is the adverb, modifying the verb "ran" by telling how the action was performed.

1124. Solve for x: 3x + 2 = 14
a) x = 3
b) x = 4
c) x = 5
d) x = 6

Answer: b) x = 4
Explanation: If we subtract 2 from both sides of the equation we get 3x = 12, then dividing both sides by 3 gives x = 4.

1125. The process by which plants use sunlight to synthesize foods with the help of carbon dioxide and water is called:
a) Photosynthesis
b) Respiration
c) Fermentation
d) Digestion

Answer: a) Photosynthesis
Explanation: Photosynthesis is the process used by plants to convert light energy, usually from the Sun, into chemical energy that can be used to fuel the plant's activities.

1126. Which word in the following sentence is a pronoun: "When Jane came to the party, she brought a gift."
a) Jane
b) Came
c) She
d) Gift

Answer: c) She
Explanation: "She" is a pronoun that refers back to "Jane".

1127. Solve the following equation for y: 2y - 3 = 11
a) y = 4
b) y = 5
c) y = 6
d) y = 7

Answer: c) y = 6
Explanation: If we add 3 to both sides of the equation we get 2y = 14, then dividing both sides by 2 gives y = 7.

1128. What is the main function of red blood cells in the human body?
a) Fight infection
b) Clot blood
c) Carry oxygen
d) Regulate body temperature

Answer: c) Carry oxygen
Explanation: Red blood cells carry oxygen from the lungs to the rest of the body, and bring carbon dioxide back to the lungs to be expelled.

1129. Identify the preposition in the following sentence: "The book is on the table."
a) The
b) Book
c) Is
d) On

Answer: d) On
Explanation: In this sentence, "on" is the preposition, indicating the relationship between the book and the table.

1130. Which of the following is an example of a gas changing into a liquid?
a) Ice melting
b) Water boiling
c) Steam condensing
d) Sugar dissolving

Answer: c) Steam condensing
Explanation: When steam, which is a gas, cools down, it condenses back into water, a liquid.

1131. Which of the following best describes the tone of the following passage: "I had the most amazing day at the amusement park. I can't wait to go back!"
a) Excited
b) Angry
c) Sad
d) Indifferent

Answer: a) Excited
Explanation: The passage indicates a positive and enthusiastic experience, suggesting an excited tone.

1132. What is the meaning of the word "benevolent" as used in the following sentence: "The benevolent king was loved by all his subjects."
a) Cruel
b) Kind
c) Jealous
d) Angry

Answer: b) Kind
Explanation: "Benevolent" is an adjective that describes someone who is kind and generous.

1133. What is the process of cell division that results in two daughter cells each having the same number and kind of chromosomes as the parent nucleus, typical of ordinary tissue growth?
a) Mitosis
b) Meiosis
c) Fusion
d) Fission

Answer: a) Mitosis
Explanation: Mitosis is the process by which a cell divides into two identical cells, each containing the same number and type of chromosomes as the original cell.

1134. Simplify the following expression: $6(2x - 3) + 4$
a) $12x - 14$
b) $12x - 18$
c) $12x + 2$
d) $12x - 22$

Answer: b) $12x - 18$
Explanation: Distributing the 6 gives 12x - 18, and then adding 4 doesn't change anything because it's not like terms with anything else in the expression.

1135. What is the primary function of the respiratory system?
a) To digest food and absorb nutrients
b) To pump and circulate blood
c) To remove waste products from the body
d) To take in oxygen and expel carbon dioxide

Answer: d) To take in oxygen and expel carbon dioxide
Explanation: The respiratory system is responsible for gas exchange—inhaling oxygen and exhaling carbon dioxide.

1136. Which of the following sentences is written in the active voice?
a) The cake was baked by John.
b) The ball was kicked by the boy.
c) Mary will be given the book by Sue.
d) Lisa ate the cookies.

Answer: d) Lisa ate the cookies. Explanation: In active voice, the subject of the sentence performs the action. In this sentence, Lisa (the subject) is performing the action of eating.

1137. Solve for x: $4x + 7 = 23$
a) $x = 3$
b) $x = 4$
c) $x = 5$
d) $x = 6$

Answer: b) $x = 4$. Explanation: If we subtract 7 from both sides, we get $4x = 16$. Then dividing both sides by 4 gives us $x = 4$.

1138. Which organ in the human body is primarily responsible for detoxification?
a) Heart
b) Kidneys
c) Liver
d) Lungs

Answer: c) Liver. Explanation: The liver is the main organ for detoxification in the body. It processes and removes toxins.

1139. What is the theme of the following passage: "Even after facing many hardships and challenges, Maria never gave up and eventually achieved her goals."
a) The importance of perseverance
b) The value of friendship
c) The effects of poverty
d) The joy of discovery

Answer: a) The importance of perseverance
Explanation: The passage emphasizes Maria's perseverance in the face of difficulties, suggesting this as the main theme.

1140. If the radius of a circle is 4 cm, what is the area of the circle? Use 3.14 for π.
a) 16π cm²
b) 8π cm²
c) 4π cm²
d) 2π cm²

Answer: a) 16π cm²
Explanation: The formula for the area of a circle is πr², where r is the radius. Substituting the given radius, we get 3.14*(4 cm)² = 16π cm².

1141. Identify the adverb in the following sentence: "The dog quickly ran across the yard."
a) Dog
b) Ran
c) Quickly
d) Yard

Answer: c) Quickly
Explanation: An adverb is a word that modifies a verb, an adjective, or another adverb. In this sentence, "quickly" modifies the verb "ran" and is therefore an adverb.

1142. The nurse must ensure the patient's consent is _____ before administering any procedure.
a) Informed
b) Assumed
c) Implied
d) Compulsory

Answer: a) Informed
Explanation: Informed consent means the patient has been fully educated about the risks, benefits, and alternatives of a procedure and agrees to proceed with it.

1143. Convert 0.875 to a fraction.
a) 7/8
b) 15/16
c) 8/7
d) 16/15

Answer: a) 7/8
Explanation: 0.875 can be converted to the fraction 7/8.

1144. Which of the following is NOT a function of the circulatory system?
a) Transporting oxygen and nutrients to the body's cells
b) Removing waste products from the body's cells
c) Producing hormones
d) Fighting infection

Answer: c) Producing hormones
Explanation: The circulatory system is responsible for transporting oxygen, nutrients, and waste products, and fighting infections. The endocrine system, not the circulatory system, is responsible for producing hormones.

1145. Which of the following words is spelled correctly?
a) Exaggerate
b) Embarrasement
c) Excelent
d) Exhilerating

Answer: a) Exaggerate
Explanation: "Exaggerate" is the correct spelling. The other words are misspelled.

1146. The process by which plants convert sunlight into chemical energy is known as what?
a) Respiration
b) Fermentation
c) Photosynthesis
d) Digestion

Answer: c) Photosynthesis
Explanation: Photosynthesis is the process by which green plants and some other organisms use sunlight to synthesize foods with the help of chlorophyll pigments.

1147. Which of the following sentences contains a simile?
a) Her eyes shone like stars.
b) The wind is a howling wolf.
c) He is a lion in battle.
d) She is the sun in my sky.

Answer: a) Her eyes shone like stars.
Explanation: A simile is a figure of speech that compares two different things using the words "like" or "as". In this case, her eyes are being compared to stars using "like".

1148. If a rectangle has a length of 7 cm and a width of 3 cm, what is its area?
a) 10 cm²
b) 21 cm²
c) 24 cm²
d) 30 cm²

Answer: b) 21 cm²
Explanation: The area of a rectangle is given by the formula length times width, so 7 cm times 3 cm equals 21 cm².

1149. Which of the following is a primary function of the skeletal system?
a) Provide support and structure to the body
b) Control body temperature
c) Filter waste from the blood
d) Aid in digestion

Answer: a) Provide support and structure to the body
Explanation: The skeletal system provides structure and support for the body, allows for movement, and protects vital organs.

1150. The word "incredulous" can best be replaced by which of the following words?
a) Unbelieving
b) Incredible
c) Indecisive
d) Indicative

Answer: a) Unbelieving. Explanation: "Incredulous" means not able or willing to believe something, so "unbelieving" is the closest synonym among the options.

1151. Solve for x: $3x + 5 = 20$
a) x = 3
b) x = 4
c) x = 5
d) x = 15

Answer: c) x = 5. Explanation: Subtracting 5 from both sides gives $3x = 15$, and then dividing both sides by 3 gives x = 5.

1152. If a word's connotation is something that is inferred, what does "connotation" mean?
a) Literal meaning
b) Dictionary definition
c) Implied or associated meaning
d) Opposite meaning

Answer: c) Implied or associated meaning
Explanation: Connotation refers to the emotional or cultural associations that a word carries beyond its literal definition.

1153. What is the chemical symbol for Iron?
a) Ir
b) In
c) Fe
d) I

Answer: c) Fe
Explanation: The chemical symbol for Iron is Fe, from its Latin name 'Ferrum'.

1154. Calculate the volume of a cube with side length 4 cm.
a) 16 cm³
b) 32 cm³
c) 64 cm³
d) 128 cm³

Answer: c) 64 cm³
Explanation: The volume of a cube is found by cubing the side length, so $4^3 = 64$ cm³.

1155. Which of the following is an example of a reflexive pronoun?
a) Himself
b) His
c) He
d) Him

Answer: a) Himself
Explanation: Reflexive pronouns are used when the subject and the object of the sentence are the same. 'Himself' is a reflexive pronoun.

1156. In the hierarchy of biological classification, what is the next level of organization above 'species'?
a) Family
b) Genus
c) Order
d) Kingdom

Answer: b) Genus
Explanation: In the hierarchy of biological classification, 'genus' is the level immediately above 'species'.

1157. A paragraph containing an overview of the main ideas to be discussed is typically found where in an essay?
a) Introduction
b) Body
c) Conclusion
d) Appendix

Answer: a) Introduction
Explanation: The introduction of an essay typically includes a brief overview or preview of the main ideas or arguments that will be discussed.

1158. If y = 5x and x = 3, what is the value of y?
a) 2
b) 8
c) 15
d) 20

Answer: c) 15
Explanation: If y = 5x and x = 3, we can substitute 3 for x in the first equation to find y = 5*3 = 15.

1159. Which of the following is NOT a characteristic of prokaryotic cells?
a) Lack of nucleus
b) Presence of cell wall
c) Presence of mitochondria
d) Typically smaller than eukaryotic cells

Answer: c) Presence of mitochondria
Explanation: Prokaryotic cells do not have organelles such as mitochondria that are enclosed within membranes. This is a characteristic of eukaryotic cells.

1160. In which part of a sentence does a predicate typically appear?
a) Beginning
b) Middle
c) End
d) Anywhere

Answer: c) End
Explanation: The predicate of a sentence typically comes after the subject, and it tells what action the subject is taking or gives more information about the subject.

1161. If 1 pound equals 16 ounces, how many ounces are there in 7 pounds?
a) 112 ounces
b) 120 ounces
c) 123 ounces
d) 130 ounces

Answer: a) 112 ounces
Explanation: If 1 pound equals 16 ounces, then 7 pounds would equal 7 * 16 = 112 ounces.

1162. Which type of bond involves the transfer of electrons from one atom to another?
a) Covalent bond
b) Ionic bond
c) Hydrogen bond
d) Metallic bond

Answer: b) Ionic bond
Explanation: Ionic bonding involves the transfer of electrons from one atom (usually a metal) to another (usually a nonmetal).

1163. What is the most precise description for the location of the adjective in a sentence?
a) Before a noun or pronoun
b) After a verb
c) Before a verb
d) After a noun or pronoun

Answer: a) Before a noun or pronoun
Explanation: Adjectives typically come before the noun or pronoun they are describing, although they can also follow the noun or pronoun in some cases.

1164. Simplify the expression: $5x - 3x + 2$.
a) $2x + 2$
b) $8x$
c) $15x + 2$
d) $2x - 2$

Answer: a) $2x + 2$
Explanation: Combining like terms gives $5x - 3x = 2x$. So, the simplified expression is $2x + 2$.

1165. Which of the following phrases best describes the main purpose of a text's title?
a) To summarize the text
b) To introduce the main idea
c) To provide supporting details
d) To state the author's viewpoint

Answer: b) To introduce the main idea
Explanation: The title of a text often provides a clue to the main idea or topic that will be covered.

1166. In humans, the type of blood is determined by which type of inheritance?
a) Co-dominance
b) Incomplete dominance
c) Complete dominance
d) Sex-linked

Answer: a) Co-dominance
Explanation: Human blood type is determined by co-dominance, where the A and B alleles are both expressed when present.

1167. Which of the following should be avoided in formal writing?
a) Use of first person
b) Passive voice
c) Slang and colloquialisms
d) All of the above

Answer: c) Slang and colloquialisms
Explanation: Formal writing should avoid the use of slang and colloquialisms, which are more appropriate for informal communication.

1168. The human body is primarily composed of which element?
a) Oxygen
b) Carbon
c) Hydrogen
d) Nitrogen

Answer: b) Carbon
Explanation: The human body is primarily composed of carbon, which forms the backbone of many important molecules in the body.

1169. Which of the following is an example of a complex sentence?
a) I enjoy reading and writing.
b) Although I enjoy reading, I like writing even more.
c) I enjoy reading; however, I like writing even more.
d) I enjoy reading, but I like writing even more.

Answer: b) Although I enjoy reading, I like writing even more.
Explanation: A complex sentence contains an independent clause and at least one dependent clause. In this case, "Although I enjoy reading" is a dependent clause, and "I like writing even more" is an independent clause.

1170. Solve the equation for x: 4x + 5 = 17.
a) x = 3
b) x = 2
c) x = 4
d) x = 5

Answer: a) x = 3
Explanation: Subtracting 5 from both sides gives 4x = 12, and dividing by 4 gives x = 3.

1171. Which of the following best describes the structure of a DNA molecule?
a) Single-stranded helix
b) Double-stranded helix
c) Triple-stranded helix
d) Quadruple-stranded helix

Answer: b) Double-stranded helix
Explanation: DNA (deoxyribonucleic acid) is a molecule that carries the genetic instructions used in growth, development, functioning, and reproduction. It is composed of two chains that coil around each other to form a double helix.

1172. The circulatory system is primarily responsible for:
a) Eliminating waste products from the body
b) Transporting oxygen and nutrients to cells
c) Controlling body temperature
d) Producing immune cells

Answer: b) Transporting oxygen and nutrients to cells. Explanation: The circulatory system's primary function is to transport oxygen, nutrients, hormones, and cellular waste products throughout the body.

1173. What is the solution to the equation 3x - 8 = 10?
a) x = 6
b) x = 5
c) x = 4
d) x = 3

Answer: a) x = 6. Explanation: To solve the equation, add 8 to both sides to get 3x = 18, then divide by 3 to find x = 6.

1174. Which of the following correctly defines an adverb?
a) A word that modifies a verb, adjective, or other adverb
b) A word that describes a noun or pronoun
c) A word that connects clauses or sentences
d) A word that shows action or state of being

Answer: a) A word that modifies a verb, adjective, or other adverb
Explanation: An adverb is a word that modifies a verb, adjective, or other adverb.

1175. What type of fat is solid at room temperature?
a) Unsaturated fat
b) Trans fat
c) Saturated fat
d) Polyunsaturated fat

Answer: c) Saturated fat
Explanation: Saturated fats are typically solid at room temperature.

1176. What is the most precise term for the "main character" in a story?
a) Antagonist
b) Protagonist
c) Secondary character
d) Foil

Answer: b) Protagonist
Explanation: The protagonist is the central character or leading figure in a story.

1177. What is the primary function of the respiratory system?
a) To circulate blood throughout the body
b) To absorb nutrients from food
c) To exchange gases with the environment
d) To filter out toxins and waste

Answer: c) To exchange gases with the environment
Explanation: The primary function of the respiratory system is to supply the blood with oxygen in order for the blood to deliver oxygen to all parts of the body.

1178. What is the solution for x in the equation $5x + 2 = 27$?
a) $x = 6$
b) $x = 5$
c) $x = 4$
d) $x = 3$

Answer: c) $x = 5$
Explanation: To solve the equation, subtract 2 from both sides to get $5x = 25$, then divide by 5 to find $x = 5$.

1179. Which one of the following words is an example of a preposition?
a) Quickly
b) Happiness
c) In
d) Run

Answer: c) In
Explanation: In this case, "in" is a preposition. Prepositions are words that show location, time, direction, cause, and manner.

1180. Which organ is primarily responsible for detoxifying chemicals and metabolizing drugs?
a) Heart
b) Liver
c) Kidney
d) Lungs

Answer: b) Liver
Explanation: The liver plays a central role in all metabolic processes in the body. In fat metabolism the liver cells break down fats and produce energy.

1181. Which of the following correctly describes the purpose of a thesis statement in an essay?
a) To provide background information
b) To summarize the main points
c) To express the main argument or claim
d) To explain the methodology

Answer: c) To express the main argument or claim
Explanation: A thesis statement expresses the main argument or claim of your essay.

1182. The passage primarily deals with:
a) The author's childhood
b) The author's favorite vacation spot
c) The author's dream job
d) The author's favorite hobby

Answer: This question requires an understanding of the passage content which is not provided here. However, in a real test scenario, the answer would be the main topic or theme of the passage.

1183. Solve for y: 3y + 4 = 25
a) y = 7
b) y = 21
c) y = 9
d) y = 3

Answer: a) y = 7
Explanation: Subtract 4 from both sides to get 3y = 21. Then divide both sides by 3 to solve for y, which is 7.

1184. Which of the following is a primary function of the skeletal system?
a) Regulating body temperature
b) Producing bile for digestion
c) Producing blood cells and storing minerals
d) Controlling the body's movement

Answer: c) Producing blood cells and storing minerals
Explanation: The skeletal system is responsible for producing blood cells and storing essential minerals.

1185. Choose the correct form of the verb: The team of researchers (is/are) working on the project.
a) is
b) are

Answer: a) is
Explanation: When a collective noun such as "team" is acting as a unit, it takes a singular verb, so "is" is the correct choice.

1186. Which substance is produced by the pancreas to regulate blood sugar levels?
a) Insulin
b) Bile
c) Pepsin
d) Gastrin

Answer: a) Insulin
Explanation: The pancreas produces insulin, which is used to regulate blood sugar levels.

1187. What is the volume of a rectangular prism with length 5 cm, width 3 cm, and height 4 cm?
a) 15 cm^3
b) 60 cm^3
c) 120 cm^3
d) 20 cm^3

Answer: b) 60 cm^3
Explanation: Volume of a rectangular prism is found by multiplying its length, width, and height. So, 5 cm * 3 cm * 4 cm = 60 cm^3.

1188. Which of the following best defines the term "osmosis"?
a) The movement of particles from an area of low concentration to an area of high concentration
b) The movement of water molecules from an area of high concentration to an area of low concentration
c) The breaking down of food particles in the stomach
d) The creation of energy in the mitochondria of cells

Answer: b) The movement of water molecules from an area of high concentration to an area of low concentration
Explanation: Osmosis is the process where water molecules move from an area of high concentration to an area of low concentration, usually through a semipermeable membrane.

1189. What is the primary function of the digestive system?
a) To circulate blood throughout the body
b) To exchange gases with the environment
c) To absorb nutrients and remove waste
d) To control body movement

Answer: c) To absorb nutrients and remove waste
Explanation: The primary function of the digestive system is to break down food, absorb nutrients, and remove waste.

1190. Which word is used to connect independent clauses?
a) Conjunction
b) Preposition
c) Adjective
d) Pronoun

Answer: a) Conjunction
Explanation: Conjunctions are words used to connect clauses or sentences or to coordinate words in the same clause.

1191. A nurse needs to administer 2.5 mg of medication per kilogram of body weight. How much medication is needed for a patient who weighs 70 kg?
a) 125 mg
b) 175 mg
c) 200 mg
d) 150 mg

Answer: b) 175 mg
Explanation: The nurse needs to administer 2.5 mg of medication per kilogram of body weight. Therefore, for a patient who weighs 70 kg, the nurse would need to administer 2.5 mg/kg * 70 kg = 175 mg of medication.

1192. The author's tone in this passage can best be described as:
a) Objective
b) Pessimistic
c) Sarcastic
d) Enthusiastic

Answer: This question requires an understanding of the passage content which is not provided here. However, in a real test scenario, the answer would be the tone or attitude of the author towards the subject.

1193. Solve for x: 2x + 3 = 17
a) x = 7
b) x = 14
c) x = 5
d) x = 9

Answer: a) x = 7
Explanation: Subtract 3 from both sides to get 2x = 14. Then divide both sides by 2 to solve for x, which is 7.

1194. Which organ is responsible for detoxification in the human body?
a) Heart
b) Brain
c) Liver
d) Kidneys

Answer: c) Liver
Explanation: The liver plays a major role in detoxification, metabolizing and excreting many harmful substances.

1195. Choose the correct preposition: She arrived ___ the meeting ___ time.
a) at / on
b) for / in
c) in / at
d) at / in

Answer: d) at / in
Explanation: "At" is the correct preposition for a specific time or event (the meeting), and "in" is the correct preposition for periods of time (on time).

1196. What role do neutrophils play in the immune system?
a) They produce antibodies
b) They destroy pathogens by phagocytosis
c) They regulate the immune response
d) They secrete toxins to kill bacteria

Answer: b) They destroy pathogens by phagocytosis
Explanation: Neutrophils are a type of white blood cell that kill pathogens primarily through the process of phagocytosis, where they engulf and destroy the pathogens.

1197. Solve: $4x^2 - 16x + 15 = 0$
a) x = 1 or x = 15
b) x = 3 or x = 5
c) x = 5 or x = 15
d) x = 3 or x = 15

Answer: b) x = 3 or x = 5
Explanation: The quadratic equation can be factored to 4(x-3)(x-5)=0, hence x = 3 or x = 5.

1198. Which hormone regulates calcium levels in the blood and bones?
a) Insulin
b) Adrenaline
c) Parathyroid hormone
d) Estrogen

Answer: c) Parathyroid hormone
Explanation: Parathyroid hormone regulates calcium levels in the body.

1199. Which of the following is not part of the cell cycle?
a) Mitosis
b) Meiosis
c) Cytokinesis
d) Interphase

Answer: b) Meiosis
Explanation: Meiosis is not part of the cell cycle. It's a separate process of cell division that results in four daughter cells each with half the number of chromosomes of the parent cell.

1200. Choose the correct pronoun: ___ is the book that I told you about.
a) These
b) This
c) That
d) Those

Answer: b) This
Explanation: "This" is the correct demonstrative pronoun to refer to something close to the speaker.

1201. A patient needs 0.5 mg/kg of a drug. If the patient weighs 80 kg, how much of the drug is needed?
a) 40 mg
b) 50 mg
c) 60 mg
d) 70 mg

Answer: a) 40 mg. Explanation: The required amount is calculated as 0.5 mg/kg x 80 kg = 40 mg.

1202. The passage primarily serves to:
a) Argue a point
b) Tell a story
c) Explain a process
d) Describe an event

Answer: This question requires an understanding of the passage content which is not provided here. However, in a real test scenario, you would identify the primary purpose of the passage.

1203. Solve for x: 5x - 7 = 18
a) x = 5
b) x = 3
c) x = 7
d) x = 4

Answer: a) x = 5. Explanation: Add 7 to both sides to get 5x = 25. Then divide both sides by 5 to solve for x, which is 5.

1204. The brain and spinal cord are components of which part of the nervous system?
a) Central Nervous System
b) Peripheral Nervous System
c) Somatic Nervous System
d) Autonomic Nervous System

Answer: a) Central Nervous System. Explanation: The central nervous system consists of the brain and spinal cord.

1205. Which of the following is an example of a coordinating conjunction?
a) But
b) If
c) Unless
d) Although

Answer: a) But
Explanation: "But" is a coordinating conjunction, used to connect words, phrases, and clauses of equal rank.

1206. In cellular respiration, glucose and oxygen yield carbon dioxide, water, and what other product?
a) Protein
b) Energy (ATP)
c) Amino acids
d) Fat

Answer: b) Energy (ATP)
Explanation: In cellular respiration, glucose and oxygen are converted into carbon dioxide, water, and energy (in the form of ATP).

1207. If f(x) = 2x + 3, what is f(4)?
a) 11
b) 12
c) 13
d) 14

Answer: a) 11
Explanation: To find f(4), substitute 4 in place of x in the function, so f(4) = 2*4 + 3 = 11.

1208. In the human body, what is the function of red blood cells?
a) Fight infection
b) Clot blood
c) Carry oxygen
d) Filter blood

Answer: c) Carry oxygen
Explanation: Red blood cells carry oxygen from the lungs to the rest of the body.

1209. If the ratio of dogs to cats in a pet store is 3 to 2 and there are 30 animals in total, how many cats are there?
a) 12
b) 15
c) 18
d) 20

Answer: a) 12
Explanation: There are 5 parts in total (3+2), and each part is equivalent to 30/5 = 6 animals. Thus, there are 6*2 = 12 cats.

1210. Choose the sentence where the word "their" is used correctly.
a) Their going to the park.
b) I'm going to their house.
c) Their is the best movie.
d) The book is their.

Answer: b) I'm going to their house.
Explanation: In this sentence, "their" is correctly used as a possessive adjective describing the house.

1211. What is the main function of the digestive system?
a) To transport nutrients
b) To break down and absorb nutrients
c) To remove waste products
d) To circulate blood

Answer: b) To break down and absorb nutrients

Well, here we are at the end of our study guide journey! We've really been through the wringer together, haven't we? From wrangling with reading structure to decoding math problems, wrestling with biology, anatomy, and chemistry, and even perfecting our English skills. And look at you now - standing tall and ready to tackle the ATI TEAS exam!

This guide has been like a friend and a coach - cheering for your dreams, recognizing it's okay to stumble, standing by your side when things got scary, and celebrating each moment of understanding. Our practice questions weren't just questions - they were tiny adventures, challenges that you took on and conquered, one by one.

You know that old saying that folks will bend over backwards for someone who supports their dreams, doesn't make a big deal about their failures, quiets their fears, backs up their hunches, and is there to say "I've got your back"? Well, this guide has been that for you. And I hope it's helped you realize you've got what it takes.

The big day of your ATI TEAS exam is almost here. A little nerve-wracking, sure, but also incredibly exciting. This is a test, but more importantly, it's a stepping stone towards the amazing healthcare career that awaits you.

So here's to you, my friend, soon-to-be healthcare superstar. This exam is just a moment in your journey, and I know you're going to rock it. Trust in what you've learned, have confidence in your abilities, and remember that each question is an opportunity to show what you're made of.

Alright, enough pep talk. It's time for you to go out there and ace that test. You've put in the hard work, you've got the knowledge, and now it's time to shine. Best of luck, my friend. You've got this!

Printed in the USA
CPSIA information can be obtained
at www.ICGtesting.com
LVHW020851100124
768131LV00080B/2610